THE COMPASSIONATE WARRIOR

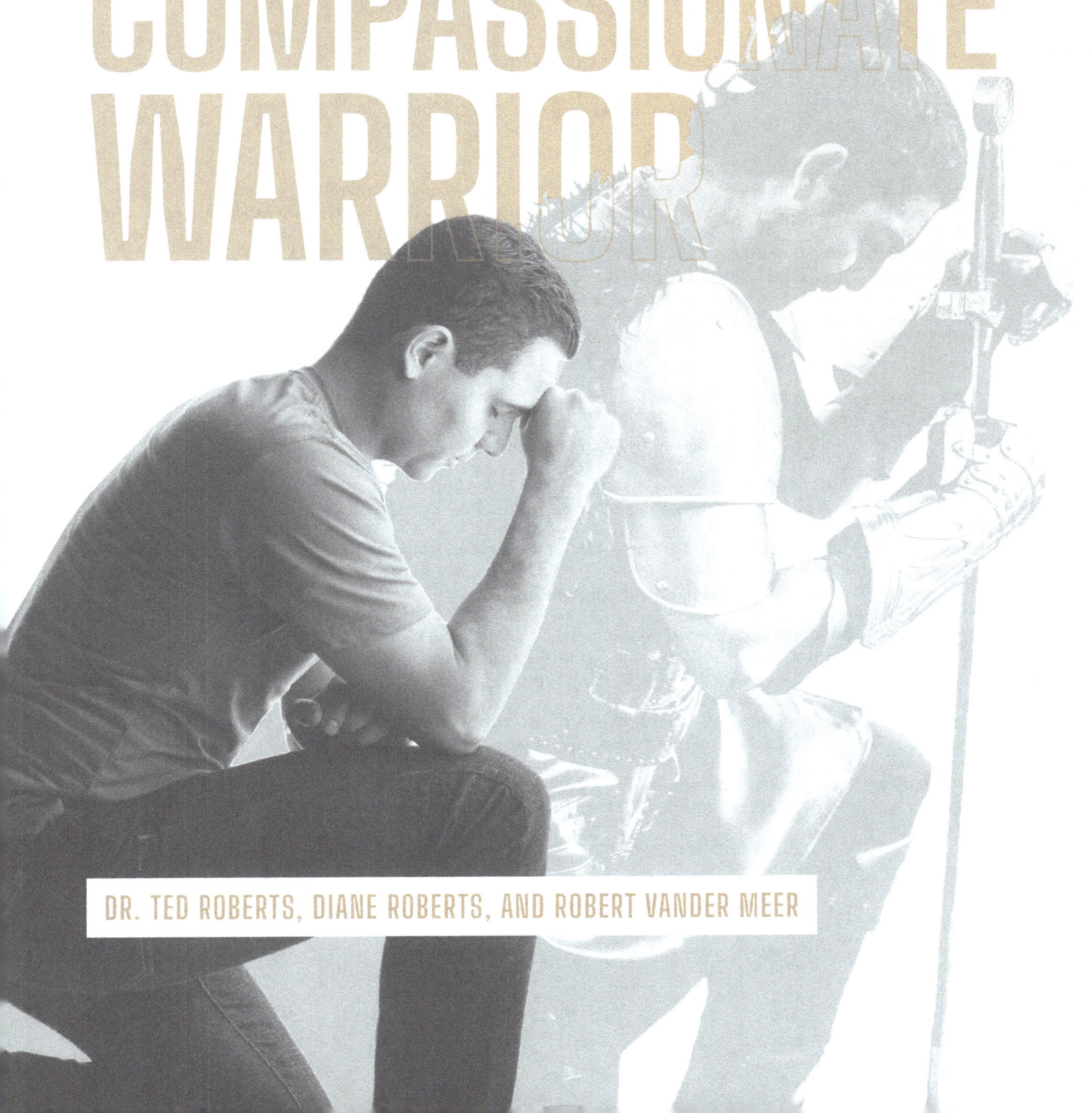

DR. TED ROBERTS, DIANE ROBERTS, AND ROBERT VANDER MEER

The Compassionate Warrior

Contributors:
Dr. Ted Roberts, Diane Roberts, Robert Vander Meer

Copyright © 2023 by Pure Desire Ministries Intl.

All rights reserved. This book or parts thereof may not be reproduced in any form, stored in a retrieval system, or transmitted in any form by any means—electronic, mechanical, photocopy, recording, or otherwise—without prior written permission of Pure Desire Ministries International, except as provided by United States of America copyright law.

Published by
Pure Desire Ministries International
886 NW Corporate Dr, Troutdale, OR 97060
www.puredesire.org | 503.489.0230

ISBN 978-1-943291-21-2

Scripture quotations marked TPT are from The Passion Translation®. Copyright © 2017, 2018, 2020 by Passion & Fire Ministries, Inc. Used by permission. All rights reserved. ThePassionTranslation.com.

Scripture quotations marked NIV taken from the Holy Bible, NEW INTERNATIONAL VERSION®, NIV® Copyright © 1973, 1978, 1984, 2011 by Biblica, Inc.® Used by permission. All rights reserved worldwide.

Scripture quotations marked NLT are taken from the Holy Bible, New Living Translation, copyright ©1996, 2004, 2007, 2013, 2015 by Tyndale House Foundation. Used by permission of Tyndale House Publishers, Inc., Carol Stream, Illinois 60188. All rights reserved.

Scripture quotations marked MSG are taken from THE MESSAGE. Copyright © by Eugene H. Peterson 1993, 1994, 1995, 1996, 2000, 2001, 2002. Used by permission of NavPress. All rights reserved. Represented by Tyndale House Publishers, Inc.

Scripture quotations marked NKJV are taken from the New King James Version®. Copyright © 1982 by Thomas Nelson. Used by permission. All rights reserved.

Scripture quotations marked NASB and NASB1995 are taken from the (NASB®) New American Standard Bible®, Copyright © 1960, 1971, 1977, 1995, 2020 by The Lockman Foundation. Used by permission. All rights reserved. lockman.org

Scripture quotations marked ESV are taken from The ESV® Bible (The Holy Bible, English Standard Version®), copyright © 2001 by Crossway, a publishing ministry of Good News Publishers. Used by permission. All rights reserved.

Scripture quotations marked AMP are taken from the Amplified® Bible (AMP), Copyright © 2015 by The Lockman Foundation. Used by permission. lockman.org

Scripture quotations marked CEV are from the Contemporary English Version Copyright © 1991, 1992, 1995 by American Bible Society. Used by Permission.

Content editing by Nick Stumbo and Heather Kolb

Copy editing by Heather Kolb

Cover design and interior design by Elisabeth Windsor

CONTENTS

VI	Dedication
VIII	Preface
XI	Group Guidelines
XII	Covenant to Contend
XIII	Memo of Understanding
XIV	Introduction: The Radical Journey Ahead

1   Stage I—Facing Evil
- 2   Chapter 1: The Divine Paradox
- 8   Chapter 2: Taking Up the Sword
- 16   Chapter 3: The Biblical Warrior

27   Stage II—Resisting the Call
- 28   Chapter 4: The "One Thing" in Life

39   Stage III—Meet Your Mentor
- 40   Chapter 5: The Warrior is Never Orphaned
- 52   Chapter 6: The Mentored Warrior Becomes the Mentor

66   Interlude: A Warning and a Blessing

69   Stage IV—A Radical Life-Altering Leap into Grace
- 70   Chapter 7: The Critical Next Step
- 78   Chapter 8: Tricky Jake—Part 1
- 86   Chapter 9: Tricky Jake—Part 2

95 Stage V—Threshold Guardians
- 96   Chapter 10: Facing Our Giants
- 104 Chapter 11: The Superhero Odyssey—Part 1
- 116 Chapter 12: The Superhero Odyssey—Part 2

129 Stage VI—The Inner Cave
- 130 Chapter 13: Only What You Take With You
- 140 Chapter 14: The Exile Within is Finally Honored

155 Stage VII—The Resurrection
- 156 Chapter 15: The Stunning Truth About the Resurrection—Part 1
- 170 Chapter 16: The Stunning Truth About the Resurrection—Part 2

185 Stage VIII—The Road Back Home
- 186 Chapter 17: I Know How this Story Ends
- 200 Chapter 18: Defining My New Normal
- 208 Chapter 19: Stumbling into Greatness

220 Conclusion: Closing Comments

234 Appendix A: Prayers for Breaking Generational Curses

238 Appendix B: Dealing with Anger

242 About the Authors

DEDICATION
FROM DR. TED ROBERTS

For me, dedications are difficult because I'm so fortunate!

I served as platoon commander in Vietnam and met Christ in the process. I also served as a fighter pilot and had the opportunity to keep some Marines on the ground alive. I returned to America and literally kissed the ground after I got off the plane. When I returned, my wife and I started a family. I had no idea how to be a dad but I somehow knew my heavenly Father would show me how to love my kids. And I have had the absolute joy of seeing my kids become some of the greatest parents on the planet!

I am so fortunate. I am blessed by God! I have the goodness of God revealed in my life through four grandchildren. The writer of Proverbs expressed it best:

> *Grandparents have the crowning glory of life: grandchildren!*
> PROVERBS 17:6 (TPT)

My grandkids have helped me hear the voice of God.

It took me over five years to write this book. I have written sixteen books and the average time involved in the writing process for each book was a maximum of about one year. So, I was confused as to when God wanted the book to be released. And did God still want me to write it? I was confused until I had breakfast with one of my grandsons, Jerratt. He responded to an email I had sent him with the following comments.

> *Hey Grandpa, saw your email. I loved it! It was beautifully crafted and thought out. I love you and don't forget, though this season may feel like the enemy is confining you. The truth is God is expanding your territory! I encourage you to write and keep writing because the season you are in right now is really tough! But that also makes it profound and beautiful. Your strength, courage, and faithfulness to God in the midst of all you are facing is inspiring me and I know it will inspire others as well. You have been called for such a time as this and I believe your story is powerful now more so than ever. Keep writing—God doesn't waste anything.*
>
> *Love You Grandpa!*

Therefore, I dedicate this book to my four awesome grandkids God has profoundly blessed me with: Jarrett, Ashley, Annie, and Ben.

PREFACE

The title of this book may puzzle some: *The Compassionate Warrior*. The title is, in a sense, a dedication to all the courageous men I have had the honor of walking beside as they battled their way to freedom.

In this preface, you have the privilege of meeting one of the bravest men I have ever known. He was committed to taking his sexual secrets to the grave. He was forever going to hide the sexual abuse that hell had orchestrated against him. Yet, when I asked him if I could use his experience as a testimony to set other men free, he didn't hesitate! This preface is dedicated to all the mighty men who God the Father doesn't hesitate to call Compassionate Warriors!

When I started my day today there was no way to know what God had in store for me. It was a normal morning. I had been wrestling with the truth of my past. I kept a secret from everyone. It was a secret I vowed NOBODY would know about—I intended to take it to my grave. In fact, before I revealed my secret to Dr. Ted, I was suicidal. I would rather die than tell this secret. I was convinced I would no longer be worthy of my wife's love; that she would leave me or divorce me. I was TERRIFIED of her finding out. When my wife and I started the process of healing with Dr. Ted and Diane, he mentioned I would be taking a polygraph test—just the thought of this put me over the top. I was terrified, not of the sexual sins of my past, but of my "secret."

Part of the healing process involved a "brainspotting" session with Dr. Ted. To say I was skeptical is not an overstatement. He sent me information about how it worked but I didn't read any of it. I decided I was going to "trust the process." I didn't need to know how it worked—I trusted Dr. Ted. We prayed and started the session. I was not prepared for the intense emotions that would come, nor the memories I had stuffed deep in my brain for 40 years.

We began by taking me back to a place I used to go to when I was struggling years ago. I described it to Dr. Ted; I was on Mt. Palomar, in southern California. I used to go camping there. I was off the beaten trail sitting by a small brook. It was a steep climb to get to. It was hidden, quiet, and soothing. The last time I was here was when I was in crisis with my father-in-law. I came to do business with God. This time, I'm here just to calm my soul. The brook is bubbling by. The birds are doing what birds do, singing to God. My blue pup tent is a few feet behind me; it's the same tent my parents gave me on my tenth birthday. The pines smell awesome. A small fire makes the air smell even better. This is my happy place: only I have been here, no one else. I breathed in the air: it's cold, very cold, I actually shivered. I was at peace. Peace with God. No stress, just happy contentment.

Dr. Ted moved the pointer to my left and, immediately, I was no longer in my happy place. He moved it slowly to my left, then up, then down. When he passed a certain spot, my heart skipped. He stopped moving the pointer. While I was staring at the pointer, my heart started racing. I was sick to my stomach, ready to retch. I closed my eyes, and I was at the place I swore I'd never go back to. I saw myself waking up 40 years ago; in a tent, at a federal campground back in the woods. I could hear laughter outside—it was my friends I had gone camping with.

Around me in the tent were a couple of empty Jack Daniel's bottles and empty beer cans. I was naked in my sleeping bag. Hungover and sick. I could hear the guys laughing, mocking me, saying how I was a "lightweight." Then I moved—I was in pain, severe pain! Shame set in immediately. What happened the night before could not have happened to me. I moved to get dressed but felt more pain! Then the realization hit me: I had been sexually abused while I was unconscious from the alcohol. They were laughing at ME! Shame set in deeper; this was my fault, not theirs, mine. The enemy whispered a lie to me that I believed for 40 years: "You are not good enough. It's your fault. Keep it a secret and no one will know."

I was weeping. Sobbing so hard I couldn't catch my breath. Dr. Ted kept reminding me to breathe and let it go. The more I cried, the harder the sobs came. Forty years of emotions came rushing out at once. I wanted to cry on my wife's shoulder, but she wasn't there. As I sobbed, I could feel the shame being lifted. I could feel the battle between the enemy and Christ fighting for my soul. I wanted to puke, run, leave, and never come back. The sobbing slowed; I caught my breath. Then it started all over again. I eventually calmed down enough for Dr. Ted to get me to focus on the pointer again.

He moved the pointer to my right, then up and down slowly. Suddenly a peace came over me. Supernaturally, it was a peace I never experienced. I was sitting at the brook in my safe place on Mt. Palomar. I was smelling the forest and the fire. Then the memory of that fateful night came to me and I was crying all over again. Slowly, just tears at first. Then the shame came back and I was weeping. While I was weeping Dr. Ted asked if I could see Christ coming down the hill toward me. I looked and Christ himself was coming down the steep bank. I didn't want to see him. I didn't want to talk with him. I actually tried to push him away, sobbing for him to leave me alone. He wouldn't leave. He sat beside me and let me cry. While I was crying, he put an arm around me and I wept on his shoulder. I cried out, "I'm not good enough" for his love. He said, "I died for you, you ARE good enough."

*I was beginning to argue with him when he handed me a gift. At first, I wouldn't accept it, but he insisted. I opened the small wooden box and in it was a beautiful ring. Handmade. It had a cross on it and on the cross an "uncut diamond." On the inside of the ring was an inscription that had my name and then the words, "**Compassionate Warrior**." He said the diamond represented me, the cross was what HE did for ME. And the inscription was HIS name for ME!*

To some, this entire experience will sound "off the wall," maybe even "made up." To be honest, I wasn't sure what I had just gone through. I wasn't sure if I could believe what happened. I didn't dare tell anyone or tell my wife about it—it was too unbelievable. When I did find the courage to tell her, we cried together. She believed me! What I DO KNOW is that my Lord touched me deeply. The healing that took place in one hour was a miracle and can only be explained as such. I can see the ring in my mind, feel it on my finger, reminding me "I AM good enough" for Christ. And, He isn't finished with me yet! "Shame" is no longer who I am. I am Christ's son!

What kind of ring do you think Christ wants to give you? I don't expect you to easily answer this question today. But by the time you finish this workbook, God will give you unique insights into the difference your life will make in this hurting and broken world! So in the space below, you can either draw an image that comes to mind now or return here later and draw a picture of the ring Father God has set aside for you.

Group Guidelines

These group guidelines were designed to create a safe environment for open and honest conversations during group meetings. Read and discuss the following guidelines as a group, including when anyone new joins the group:

Confidentiality—what is said in the group is not shared outside the group.

Self-Focus—speak only for yourself and avoid giving advice.

Limit Sharing—give everyone a chance to share.

Respect Others—let everyone find his own answers.

Regular Attendance—let your leader or co-leader know if you cannot attend a meeting.

Commitment to Accountability—make a minimum of three contacts a week. If you have relapsed in the last week, then a daily contact is recommended.

Listen Respectfully—no side conversations.

Take Ownership and Be Responsible—if you feel uncomfortable with anything, talk with your leader or co-leader, or your small group.

Stay on the Subject/Questions—watch those rabbit trails!

Homework Completion—allow 20-30 minutes per day to complete your homework. If you don't do your homework, you won't win this battle for sexual health and you will not be able to participate when the group is processing and discussing the homework.

Memo of Understanding—this document indicates you have read and understand the purpose and parameters of PD groups and the moral and ethical obligations of leaders.

Covenant to Contend (CTC)—the CTC is an open commitment of accountability which states why you have chosen to join a PD small group and what you are committed to do in order to win your battle with sexual health. At the bottom of the document you will notice a place for you and one other person to sign and date. This is a public commitment. Read the CTC and ask a member of your group to sign as a witness to your signature.

Memo of Understanding

Pure Desire Group Participants: Please read and sign this Memo of Understanding, indicating you have read and understand the purpose and parameters of Pure Desire groups and the moral and ethical obligations of leaders.

I understand that every attempt will be made to guard my anonymity and confidentiality in this group, but that anonymity and confidentiality cannot be absolutely guaranteed in a group setting.

- I realize that the group facilitator or leader cannot control the actions of others in the group.
- I realize that confidentiality is sometimes broken accidentally and without malice.

I understand that the group facilitator or leader is morally and ethically obligated to discuss with me any of the following behaviors, and that this may lead to the breaking of confidentiality and/or possibly intervention:

- I communicate anything that may be a threat to self-inflict physical harm.
- I communicate an intention to harm another person.
- I reveal ongoing sexual or physical abuse.
- I exhibit an impaired mental state.

I understand that the Pure Desire group facilitator or leader may be a mandatory reporter to authorities of sexual conduct that includes minor children, the elderly, or the disabled.

I have been advised that the consequences for communicating the above types of information may include reports to the proper authorities—the police, suicide units or children's protective agencies, as well as to any potential victims.

I further acknowledge that if I am on probation and/or parole and I engage in wrongful behavior in violation of my parole/probation, part of my healing/recovery may include notifying the appropriate authorities.

I understand this is a Christ-centered group that integrates recovery tools with the Bible and prayer, and that all members may not be of my particular church background. I realize the Bible may be discussed more (or less) than I would like it to be.

I understand this is a support group and not a therapy group and that the facilitator/leader is qualified by "life experience" and not by professional training as a therapist or counselor. The facilitator's or leader's role in this group is to create a climate where healing may occur, to support my personal work toward recovery, and to share his own experience, strength, and hope.

Name (please print) _____ **Date** _____

Signature _____

Witness: Pure Desire Group Leader Name _____

Pure Desire Group Leader Signature _____

Covenant to Contend THE COURAGEOUS FIGHT FOR HEALTHY SEXUALITY

There is a battle going on within me. As much as it pains me to admit it, that battlefield is my sexuality. I realize the outcome of this battle not only holds my life in its hands, but the lives of those I love and care for. I now choose to participate in the battle for godly character and integrity, not only for my soul but also for my family, friends, brothers and sisters in Christ, and above all else, Almighty God.

I am beginning to understand I cannot win this battle myself. I am coming to see the biblical truth that "we are members one of another." Therefore, I surrender to God's wisdom, turn to the leadership of the church, and submit myself to the process of the renewing of my mind.

THINGS I CAN DO:
- Attend a small group weekly.
- Complete the Commitment to Change and Weekly Group Check-In each week.
- God's values supersede mine; therefore, I will contend to live life on His terms instead of my own or the culture around me.
- Pay close attention to: what I look at; what I listen to; what I set my mind on.
- Take responsibility for my thoughts and actions.
- Verbally describe my feelings.
- Make contact with a group member/s at least three times between small group meetings.

I CAN ACCEPT:
- Healing is a miraculous process over time.
- Healing requires feeling the pain and learning from it.
- I am very capable of retreating back into the addictive lifestyle.
- A relapse does not stop the healing process, but it will have consequences.
- I have become skilled at lying to others and myself.
- I do not really live in isolation; my choices do affect others.
- My secrecy keeps me in bondage to my sin.

I WILL COMMIT TO:
- A willingness to change—and following through with my plans.
- Total confidentiality! I discuss only my experiences outside the group.
- Rigorous honesty with God, my small group, myself, and eventually my friends and family.
- Building my knowledge base (books, CD's, DVDs, videos, & seminars).
- Reading Scripture and praying.
- A biblical standard of sexual purity in my life.
- A goal of moving toward sobriety that is living life God's way.

Signature _____ **Date** _____

Witness _____

Now you know the structure of the group, the guidelines for group operation, and you have made a commitment to contend for your healing. This is an epic journey of transformation and we are excited for your transformation and healing. Your survival kit is intact and you are ready to go! Let the journey begin!

INTRODUCTION

The Radical Journey Ahead

The word "warrior" can strike a primal chord in the heart of a man of God. It speaks to the fact that we were never designed to just get married, pay off a mortgage, or stay single and climb the ladder, be it corporate or personal, and then be put in a hole in the ground someday. Ultimately, we were designed by God to make a difference, to put a dent in hell—in fact, to become hell's worst nightmare!

Now this is not easy to believe when all hell is breaking loose in your life. Perhaps you have found yourself trapped in the insanity of relapsing in the area of sexual health, despite the fact that you have completed a Pure Desire *Seven Pillars of Freedom* group. You may even be leading a Pure Desire group right now and also caught in the insanity of relapse—but you're unable to tell the truth to your Pure Desire group and/or your wife. It could be an out-of-control emotional response to a situation that triggers a deep sense of "not being enough," such as exploding in anger or withdrawing and shutting down, which wounds those closest to you. You realize how destructive your response can be and despite your best efforts, here you are again!

Or it could be you are facing the big 4-0, 5-0, or even 6-0, and you suddenly wake up, look in the bathroom mirror one morning, and can't remotely comprehend where all the wrinkles came from and where the time has gone. Your daily routine is built around hustling like crazy to make the next appointment, putting out the ubiquitous fires at work, taking out the trash, and walking the dog. You have been living life on autopilot. You have been totally playing defense in life which is nuts when you stop and think about it. The glaringly obvious truth is this life is 100% fatal; therefore, it doesn't make a bit of sense to shoot for survival. Life isn't meant to be survived so why not aim at hurting hell while you are here? Why not take a shot at living your life well while you're alive?

Recently, this all came to a clear point for me: I was wrestling with the fact that I had a battle just trying to walk across the room. I was a collegiate gymnast; yet there I stood with my brain sending signals to my feet but they just wouldn't move! Welcome to hand-to-hand combat with Parkinson's disease. Discouragement became my point of relapse. At times, I had an agonizing time just trying to maintain hope. Yes, God had promised me He would be with me in this battle but it felt like I was back in Vietnam, lost in what is called the "fog of war."[1] I had lost sight of the battle.

---

[1] *The fog of war refers to the uncertainty and confusion caused by the chaos of war or battle.*

Relapse will always become our lifestyle when we lose sight of the true nature of the battle. It doesn't matter if we are talking about sexual issues, emotional relapses, or quietly living life on autopilot.

It has taken me over five years to write this book. I have never wrestled so deeply with writing a book in my life. I have written or been part of developing 16 different books; so this is not my first rodeo! Why was this book such a struggle for me? The simple answer is the Holy Spirit would not leave me alone. He kept pointing out how I had superficially understood the battle. With each point of new revelation, I found myself starting all over again in the writing process. For example, I found myself recently counseling men who have led Pure Desire groups for years but were now struggling with relapse at the most fundamental level. What had I missed in training them?

The Compassionate Warrior is designed to be an in-depth answer to this question. It is intended to be a follow-up study to *Seven Pillars of Freedom*.[2] *The Compassionate Warrior* will enable you to identify areas where the enemy may have laid some emotional explosives in your life. He has strategically waited to trigger them in the days ahead so he can cripple you and regain control over your life. This workbook will also assist you in reviewing the basics of the battle which you can easily forget in the busyness of your life. This is precisely why you can find yourself caught in the insanity of relapse once again. And finally, it will open your eyes to "**The Way of the Warrior**," which is a lifelong journey God is leading you on. When you don't understand why the Holy Spirit is leading your life in a specific direction, you can end up frustrated and fighting God, which is always a losing battle. It is also critical to grasp the fact that your deepest wounds identify the most profound areas of giftedness in your lives. Therefore, it is important to understand that the areas of woundedness you battled within your Pure Desire group was part of God's call on your life. A call to be a warrior for others, not just for yourself.

It has taken me thirty years of counseling men and five years of trying to write this book to finally begin to grasp why the battle is so difficult at times.

We are at war with hell while we live this life. This is why the concept of the warrior stirs us so profoundly!

And Scripture is replete with stirring images of great battles:

- David facing Goliath
- Moses confronting an obstinate Pharaoh
- Elijah taking on 450 prophets of Baal
- The Apostle Paul being beaten within an inch of his life, then locked in a prison in Philippi, only to have God pull off an amazing jailbreak

This is the way of a Compassionate Warrior!

---

[2] Ted Roberts, *Seven Pillars of Freedom*, 5th ed. (Troutdale: Pure Desire Ministries International, 2021).

The Way of the Warrior: An Overview

There is something so stirring, yet so common to the human condition that these stories touch us at the most visceral level. Years ago, a professor named Joseph Campbell did research which uncovered the fact that myths and tales from all cultures and times share a common hero or heroine story. In other words, there is a sense of a call to a divine journey in every human heart.

Unfortunately, Joseph Campbell saw Jesus' life as just another myth, no different from Buddha or a Celtic mythical hero. He didn't comprehend that Christ was God coming down to fulfill the cry of the human heart for transcendence. Jesus was heaven's warrior to answer the dilemma of our bondage to sin that chained the heart of mankind. He paved a way through the Cross for each of us to rise up and step forth into our own heroic journey. Jesus is the ultimate Hero!

Paul makes this truth about Christ exquisitely clear in Philippians 2:6-8 (NIV):

> *Who, being in very nature God, did not consider equality with God something to be used to his own advantage; rather, he made himself nothing by taking the very nature of a servant, being made in human likeness. And being found in appearance as a man, he humbled himself by becoming obedient to death— even death on a cross!*

I absolutely love how The Passion Translation renders verse 8:

> *He humbled himself and became vulnerable, choosing to be revealed as a man and was obedient.* **He was a perfect example**, *even in his death—a criminal's death by crucifixion!*

Clearly, the mission of Jesus included a path for you and me to walk; not just to know Him but also to know the power of His Resurrection and the fellowship of His suffering.[3] But here is where I can so easily get lost in the "theological weeds." Yes, I understand that Paul declares Christ became fully man and walked on this earth so I could see how I could walk as He did. But it is nearly impossible for me to see Christ apart from His divinity, especially when we are battling with the grit and grime of relapse in our lives. However, Mr. Campbell helps us recognize the common elements found in **The Way of the Warrior** which we see throughout Scripture and literature.

Solomon gives a critical insight into every man's heart when he declares:

---

[3] Philippians 3:10.

He has made everything beautiful in its time. He has also set eternity in the human heart; yet no one can fathom what God has done from beginning to end.

ECCLESIASTES 3:11 (NIV)

As stated, the term "warrior" strikes with deep resonance in the soul of every man of God because God has set eternity in our hearts. For example, I have yet to meet a man who doesn't deeply desire to be his wife's hero. This desire is something God places there!

The common elements Campbell discovered in his work are not rooted ultimately in psychology but, interestingly enough, they are deeply embedded throughout Scripture. It is also a fascinating fact that Campbell's work serves as foundational storylines for some of today's blockbuster films. For example, George Lucas had already written two drafts of *Star Wars*[4] when he rediscovered Joseph Campbell's groundbreaking book, *The Hero With a Thousand Faces*,[5] which he had previously read in college. The blueprint of Campbell's work gave Lucas the lens he needed to bring his sprawling multifaceted universe into a focused coherent storyline. It is intriguing to note that another hugely successful movie, *The Matrix*,[6] was carefully constructed on the same blueprint.

So, what are the elements of the Hero's Journey we find so frequently delineated in Scripture and have become such a part of modern cinema? Hopefully, in answering this question, we will come to understand with new clarity our own personal journey, the struggles God is leading us through in our lives, and the battles we need to face. As Joseph Campbell eloquently expressed:

"It is by going down into the abyss that we recover the treasures of life. Where you stumble, there lies your treasure."[7]

Joseph Campbell identifies up to fourteen stages and characters in a Hero's Journey. But for our purposes, we will focus on eight stages that I call The Way of the Warrior. All eight of these stages can be clearly seen in Scripture. Here is a brief outline of the stages we will cover together in this workbook.

---

[4] George Lucas, *Star Wars: From the Adventures of Luke Skywalker* (New York: Del Rey Book, 1976).

[5] Joseph Campbell, *The Hero With A Thousand Faces* (Princeton: Princeton University Press, 1973).

[6] *The Matrix*, directed by Lana Wachowski and Lilly Wachowski (Burbank: Warner Bros, 1999), film.

[7] Diane K. Osbon, *Reflections on the Art of Living: A Joseph Campbell Companion* (New York: Harper Collins, 1991), 8, 24.

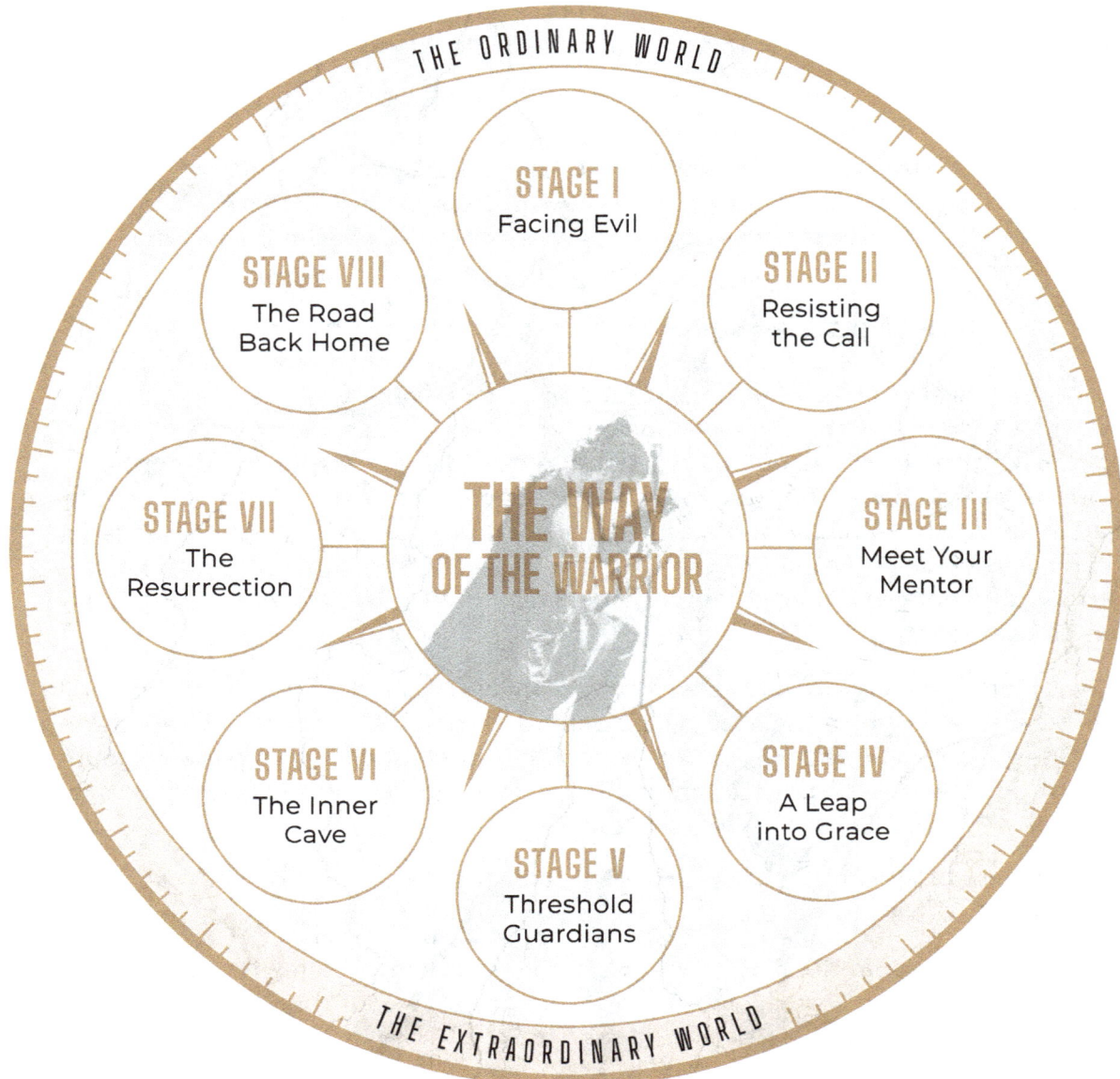

STAGE I: Facing Evil

The warrior starts off facing evil, clearly not knowing what he needs to do and, most of the time, unaware of the depth of the battle that lies ahead of him. Joseph of the Old Testament was blind to the difficult process he would need to walk through to acquire the character and capabilities to fulfill his God-given promise. In J.R.R.

Tolkien's *The Lord of the Rings*[8] Trilogy, Frodo Baggins was happy to just spend all of his days living peacefully in the Shire, unaware of the dangerous powers that were overwhelming Middle Earth.

Obviously, I am not putting the biblical story of Joseph on the same theological footing as J. R. R. Tolkien's fictional tales. Yet both Joseph and Frodo reflect common characteristics of the human struggle; and both illustrate the essence of what makes a hero a hero: **the willingness to serve others and give themselves for the greater good, even in the face of great evil around them.**

STAGE II: Resisting the Call

Those who can't or won't change begin to "live lives of quiet desperation" as Thoreau described.[9] In life, change is a constant; without change death begins to take root in our souls. Many know they should stand up and answer the call of God but, instead, they remain seated and slowly drown in mediocrity. They are frequently seated with a beer in hand, a bag of Fritos, and a remote control as they cheer on their favorite gridiron heroes in battle. The warrior, however, discovers that the path he chooses to avoid in his life ends up being totally different from the path **that chooses him**. A warrior or hero often confronts his calling or destiny in life on the very road he took to avoid the call of God. This is the hallmark of Stage II, Resisting the Call.

There is a **growing awareness** that something is deeply wrong with the hero's world. A call comes forth to change the situation and they **realize their destiny**. Frodo Baggins ends up taking the ring to Mordor, though he doesn't "know the way."[10] Moses encounters the presence of God in the burning "butane" bush.[11] It just wouldn't stop burning. He continues to ask God to "send someone else." These stories reflect different levels of resistance the warrior may have toward this journey. It will not be easy!

STAGE III: Meet Your Mentor

In stage III of our journey, we meet our mentors and, frankly, life is never the same! Mentors appear in our life under the sovereign direction of a loving God. Usually, they

---

[8] J.R.R. Tolkien, *The Lord of the Rings: The Fellowship of the Ring; The Two Towers; The Return of the King* (London: Allen & Unwin Publishing Company, 1954-1955).

[9] Robert D. Richardson, Jr., *Henry Thoreau: A Life of the Mind* (Los Angeles: University of California Press, 1986), 113.

[10] J.R.R. Tolkien, *The Lord of the Rings: The Fellowship of the Ring* (New York: Ballantine Books, 1965), 354.

[11] Exodus 3.

appear on the horizon of our life in preparation for the transition from the ordinary to the extraordinary. They are often heroes who have survived life's trials and are now passing on the gift of their knowledge and wisdom. A classic example is when Obi-Wan Kenobi gives Luke Skywalker the gift of his father's lightsaber and raises his awareness of The Force.[12] The mentor's prime objective is to impart to the apprentice life lessons and know-how learned on the battlefields of life.

Paul understood the challenge Timothy faced when he entered the pastoral ministry and spoke comforting words to his soul, *"Don't let anyone look down on you because you are young…"*[13] This mentoring comment gave him life in an impossible situation. Timothy was taking over the church as the senior pastor at Ephesus and the man he was replacing was the Apostle Paul. Talk about some tough sandals to fill! The truth is, no one successfully navigates the Hero's Journey on their own. Mentors are key to moving forward on this path.

STAGE IV: A Radical Life-Alerting Leap into Grace

Joseph Campbell once said, "Opportunities to find deeper powers within ourselves come when life seems most challenging."[14]

Joseph Campbell refers to the next phase in the warrior's way as the leap of faith or moving from the ordinary to the extraordinary in life. The hero crosses the threshold. It is precisely at this point that most folks chicken out on the journey. This leap of faith requires absolute courage and commitment for those who attempt it; they will be living far outside of their comfort zone. And as the choice is made there are no guarantees that life will be any better. The choice is the warrior's to make as he stands in the arena of his life. Or as Teddy Roosevelt expressed it—he is the one who has answered the call to strive greatly and to dare boldly.[15]

---

[12] *Star Wars: Episode IV - A New Hope*, directed by George Lucas (San Francisco: Lucasfilm, 1977), film.

[13] 1 Timothy 4:12 (NIV).

[14] Joseph Campbell Quotes. BrainyQuote.com, BrainyMedia Inc, 2023. https://www.brainyquote.com/quotes/joseph_campbell_386015.

[15] Theodore Roosevelt, "The Man in the Arena," first delivered April 23, 1910. Dickinson State University, https://www.theodorerooseveltcenter.org/Learn-About-TR/TR-Encyclopedia/Culture-and-Society/Man-in-the-Arena.aspx.

This leap of faith is Frodo leaving home and setting out on the road in *The Lord of the Rings*.[16] It's Steve Rogers receiving the super serum to become *Captain America*.[17] It is Neo's decision, in *The Matrix*,[18] to take the red pill—and discover the true nature of his reality—rather than the blue pill and stay comfortable in his false reality. It is in this leap of faith that we uncover our deepest passions and purpose in life. Or as Joseph Campbell put it, we discover "…the deeper powers within ourselves…"[19]

STAGE V: Threshold Guardians

The lessons learned in this phase are crucial to continuing the journey! **A Threshold Guardian is a blockage, a barrier, or challenge to us that we must choose to face and overcome.** This could be a villain who challenges us, a neutral character who distracts us, or even a friend who tests our desire and ability to keep moving forward. Having leapt into grace, the hero or warrior must now face that this recovery journey will happen outside of his comfort zone—it will NOT be easy!

A classic picture of dealing with a Threshold Guardian is David's confrontation with Goliath in 1 Samuel 17. This battle could have convinced David he wasn't cut out to be king, had he given into fear and run away. Instead, the victory God gave him became the building block of His future Kingdom. Or consider the U.S. military in *Captain America*,[20] as they initially send Steve Rogers to perform in stage plays to sell war bonds, rather than fight the real enemy. Both King David and Steve Rogers had to overcome these early challenges to reach their ultimate destiny. Prevailing over our Threshold Guardians will always give you and me a clearer sense of our identity in Christ.

STAGE VI: The Inner Cave

It is vital to remember, we are taking a leap into God's grace, not just a leap of faith into "whatever," or our faith in faith, or some human potential. This is what the Inner Cave is ultimately about: facing down our greatest fear or enemy, and yet discovering that God's grace is enough! In the Inner Cave, we find the stunning truth that often our greatest enemy is not in the big bad world around us but carried with us in our

---

[16] J.R.R. Tolkien, *The Lord of the Rings: The Fellowship of the Ring* (New York: Ballantine Books, 1965).

[17] *Captain America: The First Avenger*, directed by Joe Johnston (2011; Hollywood, CA: Paramount Pictures), film.

[18] *The Matrix*, directed by Lana Wachowski and Lilly Wachowski (Burbank: Warner Bros, 1999), film.

[19] Joseph Campbell Quotes, BrainyQuote.com.

[20] *Captain America: The First Avenger*, directed by Joe Johnston (2011; Hollywood, CA: Paramount Pictures), film.

own heads. One author described the darkness of the Inner Cave this way: "Generally the Shadow represents the hero's fears and unlikeable, rejected qualities: all the things we don't like about ourselves and try to project onto other people."[21]

This Inner Cave is seen in the movie *Star Wars: Episode V - The Empire Strikes Back*,[22] when young Luke Skywalker enters a cave to face down Darth Vader, only to discover his own face inside Vader's helmet. Another example of this Inner Cave is seen at the end of *the Lord of the Rings*[23] trilogy when Frodo finally has the chance to destroy the ring at Mount Doom, but then struggles with an inner voice telling him to claim the ring for himself! Discovering the strength of God's grace in our Inner Cave will give us the courage we need to complete the journey.

STAGE VII: The Resurrection

If the Inner Cave is about facing our greatest fear, then in this stage we see the final climax of the battle as the hero or warrior has his most dangerous encounter with death. In some stories or films, the hero themselves may actually experience death, while giving birth to life and hope for many, many others. This is the case for Tony Stark's *Iron Man* in the final battle with Thanos in the movie *Avengers: Endgame*.[24] In other stories, the hero will emerge from a near-death experience as a new or "re-born" character. This stage is marked by personal transformation and reward. The ultimate reward, as we will see, is being set free *for the good of others in our life*.

Paul's words in Romans 6 make it very clear that Resurrection life is something we get to experience NOW in a deeply personal experience as we walk in The Way of the Warrior. This journey is not traversed once, and then we are done. **It is a cycle we walk through again and again** as we are transformed from glory to glory.[25]

---

[21] Christopher Vogler, *The Writer's Journey: Mythic Structure for Writers*, 3rd ed. (Studio City: Michael Wiese Productions, 2007), 163.

[22] *Star Wars: Episode V - The Empire Strikes Back*, directed by Irvin Kershner (San Rafael: Lucasfilm, 1980), film.

[23] J.R.R. Tolkien, *The Lord of the Rings: The Fellowship of the Ring; The Two Towers; The Return of the King* (London: Allen & Unwin Publishing Company, 1954-1955).

[24] *Avengers: Endgame*, directed by Anthony Russo and Joe Russo (Burbank: Marvel Studios, 2019), film.

[25] 2 Corinthians 3:18 (NKJV).

STAGE VIII: The Road Back Home

This final stage is the one so many men totally miss. One of the reasons men miss this and continue to stay stuck in a cycle of relapse and shame is they never realize how the meaning of life is mysteriously revealed in the act of giving back.

Forrest Gump never missed it.[26] I love the scene where Forrest gives Bubba's mom a check, as promised, and when she sees the amount of money given to her family, she promptly faints. Also without hesitation, Forrest took in Lieutenant Dan and rescued him from a life of self-pity and anger at God. It seemed so natural for Forrest to give freely to others—to pay it forward. We also see this in the Old Testament in the story of King David. Once he sits securely on his throne in Jerusalem, he uses this opportunity to bless Mephibosheth, the lone surviving heir of his friend Jonathan. David is not only fulfilling a promise to Jonathan through his generosity, but he is also changing the entire trajectory of Mephibosheth's future!

On The Road Back Home, we will see how to create a new and lasting normal as a transformed, *Compassionate Warrior*. This stage is all about how to live in the ordinary world, but as a changed man full of confidence, peace, and purpose. This is often a return to where we started—to our marriage, family, and relationships—but never the same again!

So Are You Ready to Begin?

The Way of the Warrior involves surviving challenges, facing the Inner Cave of our deepest fears, being resurrected by the grace of God, and then returning to our starting place on the road back, as we help others on their road to freedom. We are not just traveling in a circle. We are coming full circle as we commence a new life we never thought was possible—a life that will be forever different because of the way God has led us. We are returning to the starting point with a realization of how far we have come by the grace of God. We have arrived at a point in our life we initially thought was impossible. In fact, others thought we would never end up here as well. But this is a journey God has made you for. You are His Compassionate Warrior!

Let's take this journey together. Before we dive into Stage I, take some time and reflect on the following questions. Be prepared to share your answers with your group this week.

---

[26] *Forrest Gump*, directed by Robert Zemeckis (Hollywood: Paramount Pictures, 1994), film.

What current challenges are you facing as you begin this workbook? How are these challenges the same or different from when you first started *Seven Pillars of Freedom*?

_____
_____
_____
_____
_____
_____
_____
_____
_____
_____
_____
_____
_____
_____

How are you hoping to change and grow by the end of this Compassionate Warrior study?

_____
_____
_____
_____
_____
_____
_____
_____
_____
_____
_____
_____
_____
_____

Do you see yourself as a Compassionate Warrior? Why or why not?

What is your prayer as we begin this group together? Write it out here.

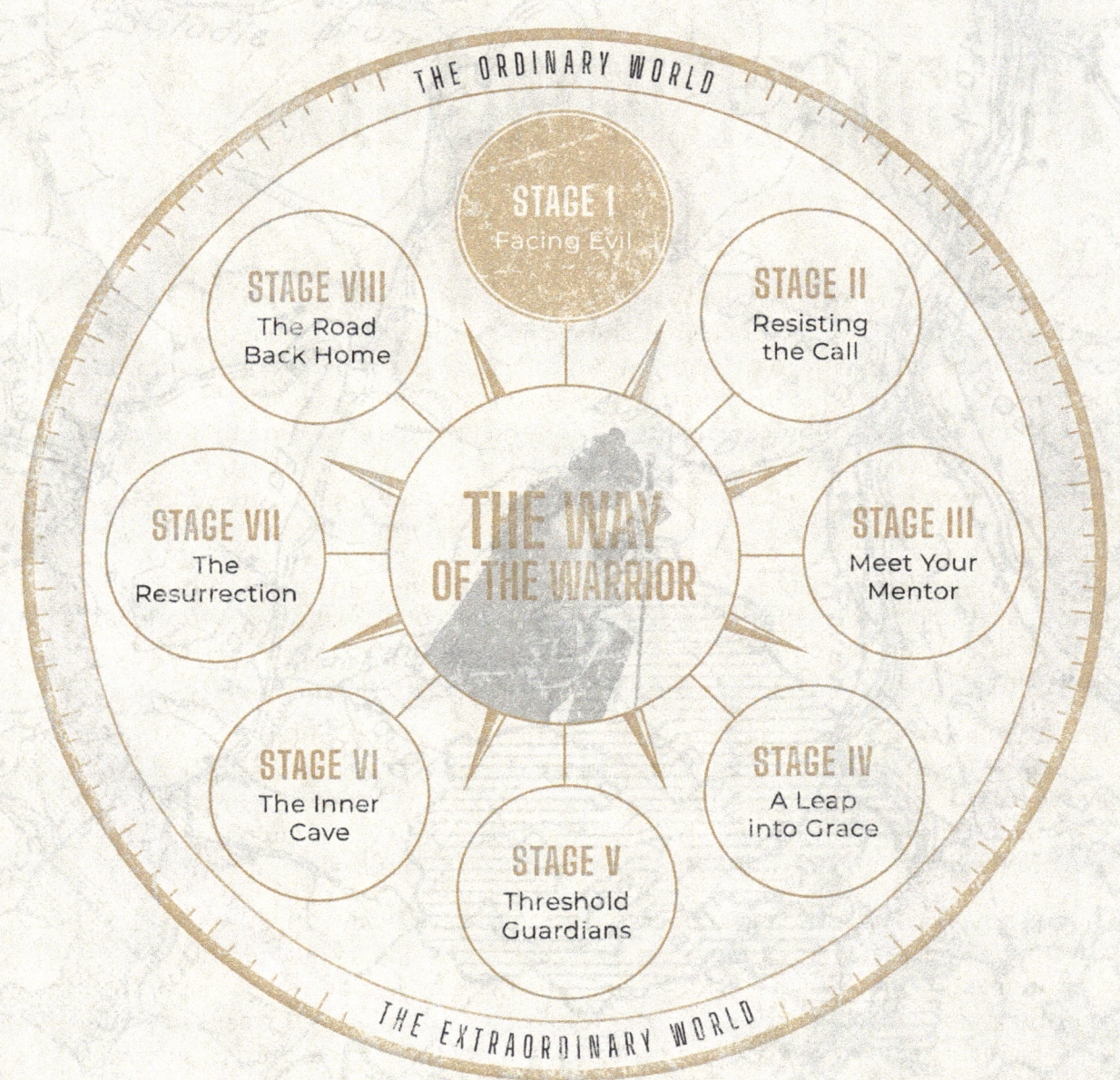

STAGE I

FACING EVIL

CHAPTER 1
THE DIVINE PARADOX

The first stage in The Way of the Warrior is to face evil. This stage is all about embracing the reality of your current situation and the truth of what it will take to overcome. Now that you have journeyed through *Seven Pillars of Freedom*, you have hopefully learned to be a man who lives in reality no matter the cost. You have identified your destructive patterns and the wounds of trauma that drive your unwanted behavior. But if you are like many men, you may find a pattern of relapse is either still present, or a new pattern is threatening to take you back to your old ways.

One thing that stands out in Scripture with unique clarity is that God is not into stagnation! This is precisely why relapses are nothing more than death on the installment plan. Sure, there may be relapses on the Hero's Journey but it was never designed by God to be a destination for you. Instead, you are designed for change. On this Hero's Journey, God wants you to be constantly discovering your full potential in Christ.

Now this can be a profound challenge if you find yourself caught in the craziness of relapse. If you have used a computer for any length of time, you have had the experience of watching your screen suddenly go crazy because of a virus that has infected the program. Or, if you have ever had the flu virus, you have had the experience of feeling like everything is going crazy in your brain and body.

In the same way, people can act in crazy, self-destructive ways because they have been infected by destructive beliefs. A destructive belief is different from a destructive thought. Beliefs reside in what the Bible calls your heart or a part of your brain known as the limbic system.[27] Biblically, your heart is the center of your emotional life; where your will and especially your beliefs reside, both positive and negative. Thoughts are ideas or concepts you have learned and are consciously aware of. Beliefs, however, usually reside at the unconscious level. They are deeper perceptions about life, safety, other people, and yourself. You will die for beliefs, but you will argue about thoughts. When a person's beliefs become infected because of destructive thinking, they can easily find themselves involved in bizarre behavior and not know why.

---

[27] Bessel van der Kolk, *The Body Keeps the Score: Brain, Mind, and Body in the Healing of Trauma* (New York: Penguin Books, 2014), 56-59.

The lengths or extremes to which an individual caught in the grips of sexual bondage will go are astonishing. This is true for many other addictive behaviors as well. It indicates the depth of infection and the degree of control the bondage has over his or her life. When it comes to addiction, we have only one option: **to access a power greater than ourselves**. We must also be willing to do things, if need be, 180-degrees differently than what we used to do. If we are not 110% committed to our recovery, more than likely, our efforts will fail and we will end up relapsing. This kind of commitment means we are willing to go to any length to not act out again. We absolutely need this depth of commitment because the path ahead is going to be extremely challenging!

This is exactly the challenge Bilbo Baggins faced in *The Hobbit*.[28] He was invited to go on a thrilling journey with a company of dwarves, but the problem Bilbo faced is that he loved his life of comfort and ease. If he wanted to go on a life-changing, grand adventure, he would have to abandon his old way of living completely—there was no halfway option! Similarly, you and I may have become comfortable with the way we do things—even in recovery. But if our current choices continue to lead us down unhealthy paths, then we also have a difficult decision to make to go all in on our recovery.

Maybe I can put it in a more personal way. Have you ever wondered why an individual in the group keeps relapsing again and again? He is doing the work and showing up for the meetings, yet he keeps falling into the same trap week after week. It has taken me a while to figure out why the insanity continues because I am so grace oriented. Now let me be quick to point out, there could be numerous causes! But after helping guys get out of bondage for almost 30 years, I have discovered there is usually one primary cause. They are not doing what Paul did.

> *But by the grace of God I am what I am, and his grace to me was not without effect. No, I worked harder than all of them—yet not I, but the grace of God that was with me.*
>
> 1 CORINTHIANS 15:10 (NIV)

The context of the passage is Paul's debate over the fact of the Resurrection but notice the nature of his lifestyle. There is this amazing dynamic in Paul realizing his next breath was a courtesy of God's grace, yet he "worked harder" than all of his adversaries! Giving 110% to the recovery process is not an option if you understand the grace of God.

Early on in this journey of grace to wholeness, one of the subtle and deadly traps is the expectation that others will applaud our efforts to walk in sexual health. This can totally knock the wind out of our best efforts because we are hoping we will be immediately forgiven for our past actions. We tend to forget how we have disappointed those closest to us again and again—and they remember.

---

[28] J.R.R. Tolkien, *The Hobbit* (New York: Ballantine Books, 1965).

Here is the hook from hell. You will have the opportunity, by the grace of God, to *eventually* restore the relationships you have betrayed. However, this will take time, much longer than you are comfortable with. It will also include a consistent effort of doing recovery work for a minimum of 30 minutes per day. Without this type of effort, your brain will not be renewed and relapse is inevitable.

So what are the beliefs that help you walk in freedom? **First, your recovery has to be more important to *you* than it is to anyone else.** Going to any length to stay clean and walk in sexual health is grounded in the fact that YOU are committed to doing whatever it takes! This means you are willing to take directions, get totally honest with yourself and others, and above all, be vulnerable and not isolate. You need to be willing to call someone when you feel like acting out, confront yourself, and pull back your own curtain of lying.

You must be willing to make a commitment to get out of your own way, give up your sexual fantasies, and let go of your desire to control others and your life. The foundation of true recovery lies in humility and surrender.

> The problem is you are pursuing healing with less passion than you pursued the addiction.

You might never have expressed it in this way. Instead, you might tell yourself, *I am not that bad, in fact I am mostly all right. It is not that big of a deal!* The bottom line is this: if you are giving less than 110%, you will continue to relapse and ultimately lose all hope.

This is one of the most subtle and deadly beliefs to get out of your head. It is so easy to tell yourself you are trying and yet not question yourself over why you are still relapsing. As we begin this first phase of our new journey, the fundamental question is: **are you more passionate about living in sexual health than you ever were about your addiction?**

NOTE: If you are not sure if your head is infected with this deadly belief, then write out your complete sexual history, including all sexual activity you have been involved in outside the marriage bed, as far back as you can remember. You may have done this work in Pillar 2 in *Seven Pillars of Freedom*.[29] If so, take out your rough draft, review it, and add any new information you left out the first time around. Use as many sheets of paper as needed. After you have written out or reviewed your history, take a few moments, pray, pause, and reflect on the results.

---

[29] Ted Roberts, *Seven Pillars of Freedom*, 5th ed. (Troutdale: Pure Desire Ministries International, 2021).

Do you recognize how crazy you were at times, risking everything for a sexual high? List your craziest moments.

How long did your addiction last? Maybe you experienced periods of sobriety, but how long have you been in a binge-purge cycle? How long have you been cycling in and out of your addiction?

In light of these facts, have you developed a greater passion to walk in sexual health than you once had for your addiction? Why or why not?

Do you think your recovery is more important to you than it is to anyone else? Why or why not?

In what areas do you need to make this healing journey more of a priority?

_____
_____
_____
_____
_____
_____
_____

What are four things you could do to develop a greater passion for sexual health?

- ▸ _____
- ▸ _____
- ▸ _____
- ▸ _____

Now, turn the four responses you wrote into an expression of surrender. Remember, if these four things are ever going to be effective in conquering your addiction, you cannot defeat the addiction on your own. **The solution begins with a paradox: victory is achieved through surrender**—surrender to the goodness of God toward you and not by trying harder.

You may be thinking: *Wait a minute! What are you saying? Are you telling me I just need to let go and let God?*

No, this is not what I'm saying.

What I am saying is that true surrender to God's goodness is an amazing paradox:

01. You will never get free unless you take total responsibility for your behavior; and out of this realization, you make a commitment to do whatever it will take to be free…period! **Nothing can be held back.**

02. If this isn't challenging enough, you are also faced with the reality that you need to make this commitment without a guaranteed outcome! You need to trust the process. For us control freaks, this is a staggering challenge! This is all totally impossible apart from the goodness of God. If your surrender is ever going to be real and authentic, you will be constantly stretched to lean into God's love for you.

Where have you held back from total surrender in your life?

What do you need to let go of today?

What beliefs do you have that keep you from leaning into God's goodness toward you? **Examples: "I will never measure up." "I can't trust anyone."**

BE PREPARED TO SHARE WITH YOUR GROUP YOUR ANSWERS TO THE QUESTIONS IN THIS CHAPTER.

CHAPTER 2
TAKING UP THE SWORD

Life is a series of transitions and how you handle the transitions will determine the depth and character of your life. Relapse can be about being stuck in a significant transition in your life—the transition from bondage to freedom, from isolation to intimacy, from hiding to living an open life, from complacency to boldly risking everything for God. You are making good progress, but it may be that you're not all the way there—not yet. You are in transition.

The significant transitions in our life are those moments when God is trying to do something deep within us. He wants to shake us free from all we have so we can be prepared for everything that is coming.

It is easy to give up things you don't want, right? These are the easy transitions. But the hard transitions are those where you are giving up something you have grown to love—like your addiction. You hate it but you also love it; which is exactly why you keep going back to it. These types of transitions are what I call "Etch-A-Moments." They are times where God is going to shake up everything that can be shaken. He will set us free from all the moments that gave us false comfort in the past so we can be ready for true comfort and everything God is preparing for us!

What are some "Etch-A-Moments" God has led you through recently or in the past?

_____
_____
_____
_____

What false comforts did you finally let go of?

_____
_____
_____
_____

Allow me to introduce you to a group of men who knew how to fight and win the battle. The Roman army ruled the known world for nearly four hundred years. There are several reasons why they were the dormant military force for so long. From a purely military perspective, there are three reasons: their discipline, their superior armament, and their ability to stand their ground. Let's take a deeper look at these reasons.

They were so well trained; they didn't panic or "go limbic" in the intensity of combat. They were able to adapt on the battlefield and find a way to defeat the enemy. The ancient battlefields were experiences of sheer brutality where opponents stood eyeball to eyeball and slugged it out. Therefore, their shoes were a critical part of their ability to stand their ground.

To start with, they wore greaves covering their knees and shins, which were made of metal so their legs could not be broken. Also, two metal spikes extended from the front of each shoe. If the soldier's sword didn't kill them, a kick from those shoes probably would. The soles of the shoes were covered with additional spikes giving the soldier an incredible ability to take a stand and nothing could move him!

In Galatians 6, the Apostle Paul describes the shoes as being "shod" which is a compound word: "hupo" meaning under and "deo" meaning to bind. These were not casual beach sandals—these were KILLER shoes!

Their discipline was legendary. For example, they would practice intense close-quarters combat everyday—both morning and evening. The swords and shields used in practice were at least twice the weight of those used in actual combat, so they were able to execute attacks in combat with tremendous speed and endurance. The main goal of the intense practice was to develop deep muscle memory at striking the enemy at his weakest points and becoming so deadly in their attacks, the enemy would be fully incapacitated and unable to respond.

Flavius Vegetius Renatus was a Roman military expert of the time. He wrote what was perhaps the single most influential military treatise in the Western world, giving us an inside look into the way they trained the Roman frontline troops of the day.

"They were taught not to cut, but to thrust their swords. The Romans would not only make a jest of those who fought with the edge of the weapon, for they found them an easy conquest. A stroke with the edges of the weapon made even with considerable force seldom resulted in kills, as the vital parts of the body are defended by both bones and armor. On the contrary, a stab, **though it penetrates but two inches, is generally fatal**."[30]

The discipline of the front-line troops of the Roman army also meant their opponents were never facing an individual on the battlefield but a wall of shields and swords

---

[30] Flavius Vegetius Renatus, *The Military Institutions of the Romans* (Westport: Greenwood Press, 1985), 20-21.

that became a killing machine. The soldiers would strike at their opponent with ruthless precision, and they would never move backward; only forward as they systematically trampled and killed their enemy.

In Ephesians 6:17, Paul is referring to these military tactics of his day as he speaks of the spiritual warfare we face in our walk with Christ. His choice of words and graphic images disclose a profound understanding of the Roman military.

> *And take the mighty razor-sharp Spirit-sword of the spoken word of God.*[31]
> EPHESIANS 6:17 (TPT)

Paul's depiction of warfare is dynamic. When describing the Spirit-sword, he uses the Greek term *machaira*; this is a double-edged sword. As mentioned, the Roman warrior would spend hours training to stab the enemy with the *machaira* instead of slashing them. In this context, Paul doesn't use the term *logos* for "word" which would refer to the written word, implying a broad general direction for our lives. It doesn't carry the meaning of dealing with the enemy by striking a precise fatal blow. Instead, Paul chose the term *rhema* which implies a specific, quickening word from the Scriptures placed in our hearts and hands by the Holy Spirit—it is personal and takes place as we experience God. Therefore, God wants to give us powerful truths to use against the enemy!

We don't need some massive 20-page document to effectively deal with attacks from the enemy in our lives. As Vegetius recorded in his history of training Roman frontline troops, all that was needed to kill the enemy was a mere two-inch stab. In the same way, one small *rhema* word from God has the power to totally devastate our adversary!

In *Seven Pillars of Freedom* we refer to this powerful weapon as a prophetic or personal promise. But it doesn't matter how powerful the weapons that God has given us, if we don't put daily effort into learning how to use them, as the Roman troops did.

In the movie *Groundhog Day*,[32] Bill Murray plays a cynical, antisocial weatherman who relives the same horrible day over and over again in the little town of Punxsutawney. It is a classic picture of a man deeply stuck in a destructive pattern. He is trapped in an endless loop until he decides to give a 110% effort to change his life. Rather than wasting the day on selfish pursuits, he eventually puts his time and effort into self-improvement and others-centeredness. Once he makes this turn, he experiences a marvelous transformation and so does everyone around him. When the

---

[31] In Greek, the word "Spirit-sword" is *machaira*, referring to a razor-sharp Roman sword used in close-quarters combat. Life.Church/YouVersion. Retrieved from https://www.bible.com/bible/1849/EPH.6.TPT.

[32] *Groundhog Day*, directed by Harold Ramis (Culver City: Columbia Pictures, 1993), film.

transformation is completed, the day finally ends and Bill Murray's character goes on with his life but in an entirely new way.

Now we may not get the opportunity for a redo of a day where we messed up—living it over and over again until we get it right. However, we do have an opportunity to improve our lives by the grace of God, one day at a time. Receiving the word of God in a personal way and then putting it into practice is how transformation occurs for us.

In Stage I of our journey, we will need to do two things:

01. Embrace the divine paradox in order to face down evil. We must take complete responsibility to give our best effort while, at the same time, completely surrender to the process by trusting God.

02. Come to a deep and heartfelt understanding of what it means to be armed by God with a *machaira*, a lethal weapon against the vicious attacks of hell.

In Hebrews 4:12, we find another description of this lethal weapon with which the Lord has equipped us:

For the word of God is alive and powerful. It is sharper than the sharpest two-edged sword, cutting between soul and spirit, between joint and marrow. It exposes our innermost thoughts and desires.

HEBREWS 4:12 (NLT)

The Greek term *distomos* describes a two-edged sword; it literally means "two-mouthed." The author of Hebrews uses this to describe a two-step process: first, the word comes out of the mouth of God to you; and second, you then turn and speak it into the face of hell. At this moment, it becomes alive and powerful, cutting against the forces of hell aligned against you, your family, your ministry, your finances, or your body.

To understand the power of this double-edged, two-mouthed sword, consider what happened to Jesus. In the book of Mark, we find the depiction of Christ's baptism by John. It is a stunning, special effects event in the kingdom of God. As Jesus came up out of the water, the heavens were "split apart" which is an insight Mark gives us describing the intensity of the moment.[33] This is immediately followed by the descent of God the Holy Spirit upon the Son; and Father God declaring openly that Jesus is His Son, with whom He is well pleased.

It is critical that we realize all of this takes place well before Christ had done a single miracle. The love of the Father for the Son had nothing to do with his performance! In this extraordinary moment, God the Father proclaimed that the Son belonged—he was loved by the Father and the Father praised him.

---

[33] Mark 1:9-11 (LEB).

This reality needs to be present in all of our lives if we are to have a strong sense of our identity. If we are ever going to know who we are and who we are not, like Jesus, we need to have the Father speak over us and to us! Once we hear the Father's words of delight over us and for us, no one can take this away from us. Therefore, it is essential for us to learn how to effectively respond to God's *rhema* word to us.

Mark's rendition of the baptism gives us another unique insight into the Holy Spirit's role in this critical time in Christ's life. It says, "Immediately the Holy Spirit **forced him out into the wilderness**."[34] As Christ stepped out of the waters of baptism and that glorious moment of basking in the words of his Father's approval, he was literally driven into the searing heat and loneliness of the Judean desert. Both Matthew and Luke describe the Spirit as leading him; they didn't use such forceful terms. We can't know exactly what was behind Mark's choice of words but it definitely means this time of testing was God-ordained and it was part of Jesus' preparation.

In Luke, we find a subtle statement which implies the purpose of the temptation.[35] In Luke 4:1, we read that Christ was full of the Holy Spirit as the Spirit led him into open confrontation with Satan in the wilderness. But in verse 14, we find the following change had taken place: "Jesus returned to Galilee **in the power of the Holy Spirit**." This was the launching point of Jesus' ministry. Luke is emphasizing how all the miracles that would flow from Jesus were a result of the Holy Spirit's power flowing through him. And the implication is that the Holy Spirit's power can flow through our lives as well, if we learn to face the challenge of hell's work in our world.

In the abbreviated version of the baptism in Mark, there are **two dynamics of God's word** that stand out with clarity. First, Satan's attack against Jesus was personal and very intense in contradiction to God's word! This is clear when Satan continues to say, "If you are the Son of God..." The use of the word "If..." actually carries the meaning of "since."[36] The Devil is not directly attacking Christ's identity but instead is attempting to misdirect his mission. He is basically saying to Jesus, "Since you are good with God, why don't you do what you want to do? Come on, you don't have to put up with this kind of pain."

In this subtle and deadly attack, you see the essence of all sin. It is grounded in the belief that God isn't ultimately dedicated to our good. This false belief says that if we give Him complete control, we will be miserable. Why the Holy Spirit specifically led Jesus into the wilderness now becomes obvious. No one has a struggle believing in the goodness of God when everything is going our way. But when everything in our

---

[34] Mark 1:12 (AMP).

[35] Only in Luke does Jesus "set his face toward Jerusalem" (9:51 EXB). In Luke 13:33 we find the statement, "Surely no prophet can die outside of Jerusalem." Therefore it is appropriate that the temptation scenes reach a crescendo there.

[36] Robert K. Johnston, Robert L. Hubbard Jr., and W. Ward Gasque, *Understanding the Bible Commentary*, New Testament, Mark (Grand Rapids: Baker Publishing Group, 2011), 508.

life goes sideways and all hell breaks loose—well, this is another story! Although we may feel a sense of shame and guilt if we are viewing pornography or having a "little fling" with a coworker, at some point, we will find ourselves at a deeper crossroads where we say to ourselves, *If I repent and obey God, I am going to miss out! I need to be happy!* This is the justification we use. **Sin always begins with the character assassination of God! The original sin was about knowing God yet believing He couldn't be trusted.**

We think, *If I can't trust God then the only person I can trust is **myself**. I am alone. No one cares. I have to take care of myself.* These are vows we can construct out of the painful moments we may encounter in life. This is the same lie the serpent fed Adam and Eve. This is really the most fundamental temptation there has ever been in our broken world. But the gospel writer, Luke, refers to Jesus as "...the son of Adam, the son of God."[37] Luke is drawing a stunning picture of Christ, who not only suffered for us in the Judean wilderness but also on the Cross. He took to himself all of the collective Adam's who have ever lived. All our sin, shame, and guilt.

Man takes this lie into his heart and, out of his fear of missing the good things in life, asserts himself against God. He puts himself where God deserves to be. And God sacrifices Himself for man and puts Himself where man deserves to be. Man claims prerogatives that belong to God, and yet God accepts penalties that belong to man alone!

In order to move ahead in this journey, we must choose to believe the word of God that is spoken to us, just as Jesus did at his baptism. Satan will do whatever he can to cause us to question this word but, like the Roman army, we must stand firm with our feet planted securely in God's truth spoken to us.

Before we get to the second dynamic of God's word in Jesus' baptism story, take a moment to wrestle with the following questions:

> Have you ever found yourself struggling with believing God wasn't working on your behalf? Describe this struggle.

---

[37] Luke 3:38 (ESV).

> During the struggle you described, what were you facing that caused you to doubt God's goodness?

> What happened that enabled you to start trusting God?

The second dynamic of God's word that stands out when reading the conflict between Christ and Satan is how **Jesus uses the words of God as His weapon for victory**. All of Jesus' responses to Satan are quotes from Deuteronomy. The three temptations Christ faced were the exact same temptations Israel had faced in the wilderness and failed. Luke is underlining how the last Adam—Jesus—had totally won victory over the very issues the first Adam completely collapsed under.[38] In every one of Christ's responses to Satan, "It is written…" is, in essence, a counter punch. It wasn't simply a Bible memory contest. Jesus wasn't quoting a Bible verse he liked. The enemy's primary attacks against us will not just be intellectual. The major battlefield will **always engage our emotions**. And remember, our limbic system is reprogrammed by new experiences, not just new information.

Remember the special effects show heaven presented in honor of the Son? The heavens were torn apart, the Holy Spirit descended like a dove, and the booming voice of the Father openly declaring His delight in the Son. This was an incredible emotional moment for both heaven and earth! This was the emotional power behind each of the verses Jesus quoted. It was the double-edged *machaira* sword piercing the lies of hell. The words of Christ were like the precision strikes of a skilled warrior penetrating the vulnerable parts of the enemy's attack, immediately neutralizing his best efforts. Therefore, the only thing the enemy could do was retreat and look for a better time to take his best shot.

When I read Luke 4:1-13 describing the battle between Satan and Jesus, I realized, if Christ needed a promise from God to deal with the attacks from Satan concerning his identity, **how much more I need one**!

---

[38] Johnston, et al., *Understanding the Bible Commentary*, 510-512.

Has God given you a personal promise that stopped the enemy in his tracks? What was the emotional experience or encounter you had with God? Who did He say you are?

_____
_____
_____
_____

If you are having difficulty identifying this kind of encounter with God, answer the following questions as a pathway to discover your personal promises. (You may also refer back to Pillar 6, Lesson 4 in *Seven Pillars of Freedom* to see the promises you wrote in that lesson.)

1. Identify 2-3 times in your life when you felt God was particularly near to you. What was happening in your life?

_____
_____
_____
_____

2. What are 2-3 of your favorite passages of Scripture? Why do these passages have such strong personal meaning for you?

_____
_____
_____

3. What has happened in your life to convince you that God is real and truly loves you?

_____
_____
_____
_____

Share these answers with your group and see if together you can begin to identify some of God's personal promises to you!

BE PREPARED TO SHARE WITH YOUR GROUP YOUR ANSWERS TO THE QUESTIONS IN THIS CHAPTER.

CHAPTER 3
THE BIBLICAL WARRIOR

If we are ever going to fully face evil and take The Way of the Warrior path, we must understand that we have been called into this adventure by God. He has called you and me to be a biblical warrior and this call of God on our lives will become our motivation to take action. As we embrace this call, our mission with God can truly begin. In this chapter, we will see what it means to embrace God's call to be a biblical warrior.

After seeing the original *Top Gun*[39] movie in the 1980s, I can remember getting more and more frustrated as my friends turned to me with excitement written all over their faces, asking, "Wow, did you ever do that?" I tried to explain to my awestruck friends that the movie was more like a comic book. It had little, if any, correlation to the reality of flying an actual fighter aircraft and the insane intensity of a dog fight. For example, the "hard deck" in the movie was supposedly set at 10,000 feet. Yet, at times, you saw the mountain peaks towering over the aircraft. The training must have taken place in the Himalayas!

Yet, the opening scene—the steam rising off the carrier deck as the deck hands lean against the wind—brought back a flood of memories; memories of personally experiencing the deadly ballet of tightly coordinated movements of men and machines on a carrier deck. It is one of the most dangerous places in the world to work and, at the same time, it is incredibly exciting! The classic example is the "shooter" with his hand raised overhead, fingers rapidly circling as he signaled for the pilot on the catapult to bring his aircraft up to maximum power.[40] This is followed by a dramatic forward lunge, as the wing of the aircraft slices through the air, screaming overhead, like a giant samurai sword. This scene brought back the incredible experience and adrenaline rush of being thrown off the front end of an aircraft carrier! But I was deeply frustrated by how Hollywood's first *Top Gun*[41] movie had taken the challenge of being a Naval Aviator and turned it into a comic book character.

---

[39] *Top Gun*, directed by Tony Scott (Hollywood: Paramount Pictures, 1986), film.

[40] America's Navy, *Catapult Officer*, https://www.navy.com/careers/catapult-officer.

[41] *Top Gun*.

(Fortunately, the newest movie, *Top Gun: Maverick*[42] was fairly accurate in the presentation of the challenging task of taking out a highly defended target. That is until Tom Cruise took out several Soviet SU-57, which is a fifth gen fighter—in other words, it was the top-of-the-line Soviet fighter! The crazy thing about the final scenes is how Tom Cruise pulls this amazing feat of airmanship while flying an old beat-up and falling apart F-14! But I digress…)

Today, I am even more irritated by the way in which the concept of a warrior has been so distorted by our culture. The biblical picture of a warrior is so radical; in a way, I can almost grasp how it is so easily misunderstood by our world. It is paramount that we come to an understanding of the richness and incredible challenge of becoming a "warrior" from a biblical perspective. And here's why: if we don't know who God has called us to be, we can so easily end up being someone else and never become the biblical warrior God has called us to become.

This is huge because **if you have ever struggled with sexual bondage in your life, then you are called to be a warrior for those who are still trapped by hell**! If you don't understand "The Way of the Warrior" and can't see where you are headed in life, you can easily become confused by what is happening in your life or end up deeply discouraged or mad at God! Therefore, understanding the biblical picture of a warrior is not an option for you. For example, you will never integrate the disciplines of real freedom in your life, if you don't have a clear picture of what this looks like.

I have seen so many young men distracted by trying to imitate Steve McQueen, or *Jason Bourne*[43] (played by Matt Damon), or *Rocky*[44] (played by Sylvester Stalone), or some favorite athlete, or even their abusive father. These men may play the role of being a warrior but becoming a biblical warrior involves a whole other level of challenge!

You may be wondering, *Where can we find a description of such a radical kind of man?* Would you believe in the Bible? And it involves one of my closest friends in Scripture, David.

When I find myself going through a tough time, which is quite often, like David, I can make some really dumb choices in life. When I am struggling in life, I will slowly read through the Psalms of David. In the process, I am being drawn back into an intimate relationship with God. It's awesome! The thing that intimidates the enemy more than anything else is our intimacy with God. Through the years of studying David's life, I realized he was made great by the men who served him. There were three men in particular and they were called the leaders of David's Mighty Men. Scripture reveals an exquisite picture of biblical warriors set as a stunning backdrop to David's life.

---

[42] *Top Gun: Maverick*, directed by Joseph Kosinski (Hollywood: Paramount Pictures, 2022), film.

[43] *The Bourne Identity*, directed by Doug Liman (Universal City: Universal Pictures, 2002), film.

[44] *Rocky*, directed by John G. Avildsen (Los Angeles: Chartoff-Winkler Productions, 1976), film.

These are the names of David's mightiest warriors. The first was Jashobeam the Hacmonite, who was leader of the Three—the three mightiest warriors among David's men. He once used his spear to kill 800 enemy warriors in a single battle.

Next in rank among the Three was Eleazar son of Dodai, a descendant of Ahoah. Once Eleazar and David stood together against the Philistines when the entire Israelite army had fled. He killed Philistines until his hand was too tired to lift his sword, and the Lord gave him a great victory that day. The rest of the army did not return until it was time to collect the plunder!

Next in rank was Shammah son of Agee from Harar. One time the Philistines gathered at Lehi and attacked the Israelites in a field full of lentils. The Israelite army fled, but Shammah held his ground in the middle of the field and beat back the Philistines. So the Lord brought about a great victory.

2 SAMUEL 23:8-12 (NLT)

Jashobeam's actions sound like some contemporary "superhero" from a Marvel comic book. It is fascinating to note that the term "superhero" came into usage barely 80 years ago. With the creation of Superman, by Jerry Siegel and Joe Shuster, we had the development of the realm of adventure science fiction.[45] The number of superhero movies has grown exponentially in recent years. Both Marvel and DC Comics have released movie after movie with superheroes inspired from their comic book series.

Why is there such a recent fascination with superheroes? I mean, when you think of a mighty hero, they have rippling muscles, incredible courage, and are invincible in battle. Yet they all have one fatal weakness. When thinking about superheroes, Superman usually comes to mind; but if you stop and think for a minute, you realize this story actually has a long, long history. It's not just 80 years old. Remember Achilles and his heel (which was his weakness; his kryptonite)? The ancient myth tells the story of a great hero, Achilles. His mother dipped him in the River Styx when he was a child and, as a result, he became invincible in battle—except for one spot: the heel by which she held him.

My point is that this isn't just a recent fad or fascination. I am convinced, deep in the heart of every man there is a **God-given** desire to make a difference in this world. This is exactly why Joseph Campbell's research uncovered the Hero's Journey across a multiplicity of cultures and countries. The superhero has become such a fascination in the films of our day because we have **substituted the power of God** with science fiction and fantasy. There are some deeply personal reasons for this present day fad which we will look at in later chapters.

---

[45] Alyssa Smith, *Rise of the Superhero: From the Golden Age to the Silver Screen* (New York: Life Books, 2017), 6.

As we look back at Scripture, an interesting question to ask is: "Where did these mighty men begin their journey? The answer is found in 1 Samuel 22:2:

All those who were in distress or in debt or discontented gathered around him, and he became their commander. About four hundred men were with him.
1 SAMUEL 22:2 (NIV)

This was the original "hole in the wall" gang. David was hiding in a cave, from the homicidal maniac King Saul, with 400 guys who were broke, busted, and disgusted. But why were they drawn to him? And what turned this bunch of losers into an awesome fighting force of mighty men?

These men were drawn to and transformed by David's God inspired dream! And it worked both ways; without his mighty men, David would have just been another fugitive with a pipe dream hiding in a cave. Warrior's dreams don't just occur in isolation. These types of dreams always stand on the shoulders of those who have gone before us.

My dream of leading a large, healing church was a result of my time spent serving with a pastor named Butch Plummer. I remember when I first encountered Butch. He was asked to be a speaker at the Bible College where I had found myself serving as a professor. It was one of the worst times of my life. I was slowly dying spiritually. As part of the facility, I was seated in the front row. My head was down because I knew this was going to be another boring exercise in religiosity. First of all, I noticed his shoes; he was wearing these shiny, metal toe capped shoes! He had a maroon colored jacket with a pink scarf and a pair of tinted glasses with the word "Shepherd" in diamonds on one lens. I was thinking, *This guy isn't even saved!* But when he opened his mouth, I heard about the love of God like I had never heard it before. I eventually ended up serving on his staff. Once after a service, I remember him holding a broken and hurting man in his arms with tears streaming down his face. It was then I cried out to God, "I want to be a pastor like Butch, Lord."

Our dreams predate us. They were born before we even arrived on the scene. And these God-given dreams will make a difference long after we are gone.

> Whose shoulders are you standing on with respect to your God-given dreams? Who inspired you to pursue the dreams you are now pursuing?

_____
_____
_____
_____
_____

Jashobeam raised his spear against 800 adversaries. These are impossible odds: 800-to-1! Take out one guy and there are 799 waiting in line behind him to take you down.

God absolutely loves these odds. Remember when He reduced Gideon's army by 99% down to only 300 men? Gideon was facing an army of Midianites, Amalekites, and other eastern peoples which Scripture describes, as so large "it was impossible to count the men and their camels."[46] God also chose an old geezer named Moses, who had a stick and a stutter, to take on the most powerful army in the world at that time. The reason God delights in these odds is, as God said to Gideon, *"So that you will not be able to say your own strength saved you!"*[47] People who are dreaming the dreams of God will always face impossible odds.

> When was the last time you attempted something so audacious for God, if He didn't show up you were toast? When was the last time you faced impossible odds to follow your God-given dream?

In David's mighty warriors, we can see three "Cs" of a warrior. Jashobeam was a classic example of **courage**. Courage is non-negotiable for a warrior leader. Colonel Wesley L. Fox, who earned the Medal of Honor as a rifle company commander in Vietnam, as he cogently observed, "The only character trait that I would rate over integrity is courage, because without courage to hold the line of truth, one will lie."[48]

The second warrior, Eleazar, fought until his hand was too tired to lift his sword any longer. The NIV translation of verse 10 says, "...*his hand grew tired and froze to the sword*."[49] No one could outlast Eleazar. You see, he defeated his foes long before they ever met on the battlefield. The battle is ultimately won in the weight room not on game day or as Muhammad Ali expressed it, "I hated every minute of training, but I said, 'Don't quit. Suffer now and live the rest of your life as a champion.'"[50]

---

[46] Judges 6:5 (NIRV).

[47] Judges 7:2 (NIV) paraphrase.

[48] Wesley Lee Fox, *Six Essential Elements of Leadership: Marine Corps Wisdom of a Medal of Honor Recipient* (Annapolis: Naval Institute Press, 2011), 67.

[49] 2 Samuel 23:10 (NIV).

[50] Muhammad Ali Quote, Goodreads, Inc., https://www.goodreads.com/author/quotes/46261.Muhammad_Al.

Eleazar was not just **committed** to his personal victory. Eleazar was committed to David. Notice the phrase in verse 9: "...*Eleazar and David stood together against the Philistines...*"[51] And apparently they were alone on the battlefield facing the Philistines: "*The rest of the army did not return until it was time to collect the plunder!*"[52] I can picture these two warriors standing back to back taking out the enemy!

It was a gripping illustration of courage and commitment together to a God-given dream.

> When have you had the joy of winning a great victory with a close friend as you both fought for a God-given dream?

> If this hasn't happened in your life yet, where do you dream of it happening in the future?

The final champion of the three, Shammah, held his ground in the middle of the field and beat back the Philistines when the entire army of Israel had deserted him! And it was just a field of lentils, one of the most common crops of the day historically going all the way back to the time of Jacob.[53] Shammah's stand to defend something that was so common powerfully illustrates the depth of his **character**. He obviously took a stance based on his inner values not on a potential for personal rewards.

- Jashobeam was an example of **Courage**.
- Eleazar was an example of **Commitment**.
- Shammah was an example of **Character**.

All three of these men had a similar heart: they would never tap out in life!

---

[51] 2 Samuel 23:9 (NLT).

[52] 2 Samuel 23:10 (NLT).

[53] Merrill Chapin Tenney, *The Zondervan Pictorial Encyclopedia of the Bible*, Volume 3 (Grand Rapids: Zondervan Publishing House, 1975), 909.

But their next decision in combat raised their leadership to the radical biblical level and helps us see a powerful fourth "C" of leadership:

> *David had a sudden craving and said, "Would I ever like a drink of water from the well at the gate of Bethlehem!" So the Three penetrated the Philistine lines, drew water from the well at the gate of Bethlehem, and brought it back to David. But David wouldn't drink it; he poured it out as an offering to GOD, saying, "There is no way, GOD, that I'll drink this! This isn't mere water, it's their life-blood—they risked their very lives to bring it!"*
>
> 2 SAMUEL 23:16-17 (MSG)

David expressed the desire of his heart for a drink of water from the well he knew as a boy. He had probably gone there frequently during the harvest season to receive a refreshing drink of water. These three mighty men cared so deeply for their commander, they marched the twelve miles fighting their way through the Philistine lines to respond to the longing of David's heart. David also profoundly cared for his men as well and he understood the great risk they had taken. So he poured out the water as an offering to the Lord; he resisted the temptation to pull rank.

This is completely counter to great warrior cultures of the past and present. The Japanese warrior culture of Bushido was shame based, which required those who were seen as cowards to commit ritual suicide. The mighty Spartans of Thermopylae fame were also a deeply shame-based warrior culture (remember the movie 300?[54]). The maidens of Sparta were taught songs of ridicule to humiliate any young man who displayed a lack of courage on the battlefield.[55] In a shame-based culture, saving "face" is everything. All that matters is what the community believes about you. The warrior advancing into battle is more afraid of disgrace in the eyes of his community than of the spears and swords of the enemy. The typical warrior culture down through the centuries has motivated the individual to face his fear in battle through the greater fear of public shame and humiliation.

But remember, this shame will deeply drive your addictive behavior unless you learn to view yourself based on what God thinks about you instead of the fear of what others think about you. Until you experience this radical perspective change, you will never get free from the insane cycle of relapse. **In David's mighty men you see the most critical factor in leadership and the answer to shame—caring.**

Colonel Wesley L. Fox's words are so profound at this point: "Care is a personal commitment to people and the things those people value. Care for one's followers is in my opinion the number one essential element of leadership. When followers realize that their leader doesn't really care about them, he is no longer their leader.

---

[54] *300*, directed by Zack Snyder (Burbank: Warner Bros., 2006), film.
[55] Steven Pressfield, *The Warrior Ethos* (New York: Black Irish Entertainment, LLC, 2011), 22.

He is only a figurehead."[56]

Then Colonel Fox's words plow even deeper into the challenge of leadership: "Marine leaders are known for the care of their men, but how do they handle the task of sending them forward into battle?"[57] The Colonel spends the rest of the chapter wrestling with the battlefield implications of caring and leading.

Now you are probably not going to be facing a military battlefield anytime soon but your ability to care for your wife, children, and friends is a true mark of how effective of a leader you are.

A biblical warrior is a man who displays all four Cs of leadership, not just for himself but primarily for the good of others: **Courage, Commitment, Character, and Care**. We must develop all four of these areas as we walk in The Way of the Warrior and live a transformed life!

> How are you doing with the four Cs of leadership? On a scale of 1 to 10, score yourself in each of these areas. If you're married and/or have kids, ask your wife to rate you and your kids to do the same, especially if they are teens.

COURAGE:

Weak and fearful — Bold in the Lord

1　　2　　3　　4　　5

COMMITMENT:

Flaky and unreliable — I'm all in

1　　2　　3　　4　　5

CHARACTER:

Inconsistent — Rock solid

1　　2　　3　　4　　5

---

[56] Wesley Lee Fox, *Six Essential Elements of Leadership*, 53.

[57] Wesley Lee Fox, *Six Essential Elements of Leadership*, 53.

CARE:

| Numb and disassociated | | | | Others feel deeply cared for |

1   2   3   4   5

YOUR WIFE'S (OR GIRLFRIEND'S) RATING OF YOU:

| Completely self-focused | | | | My husband cares deeply for me |

1   2   3   4   5

YOUR KID'S (OR FAMILY MEMBER'S) RATING OF YOU:

| He doesn't care | | | | He cares about me |

1   2   3   4   5

What did you learn about yourself?

_____
_____
_____
_____
_____
_____
_____
_____
_____
_____

What are your areas of strength?

In what areas can you improve? If you are bold enough to do it, ask your wife; or if you are single, ask your girlfriend or close friend.

Based on what you've learned so far, how is it helping you become a Compassionate Warrior? Be specific in your answer.

BE PREPARED TO SHARE WITH YOUR GROUP YOUR ANSWERS TO THE QUESTIONS IN THIS CHAPTER.

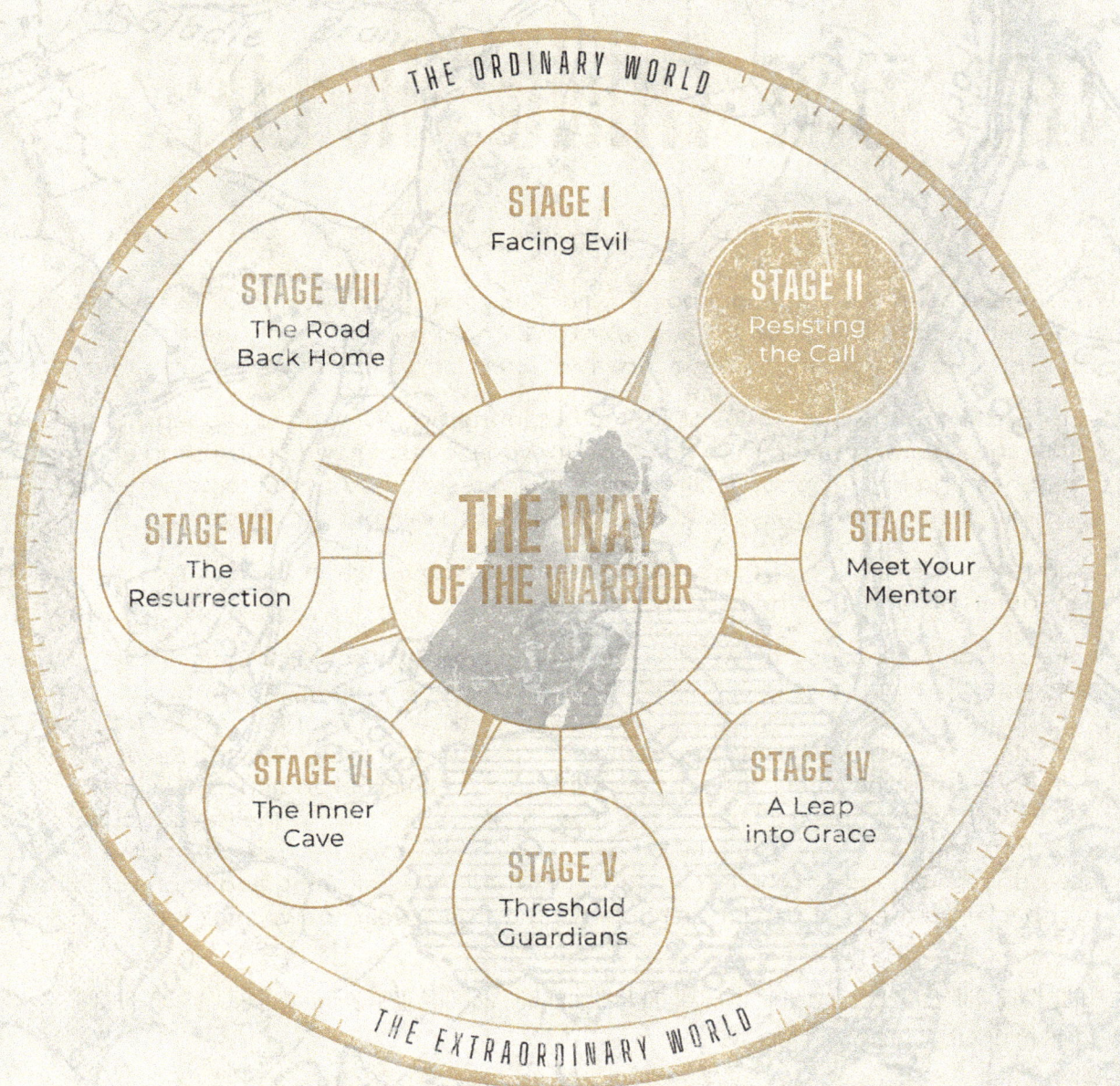

STAGE II
RESISTING THE CALL

CHAPTER 4
THE "ONE THING" IN LIFE

We all have been there at some point in our life: when God is asking us to say "yes" to an adventure that will be exciting and, at the same time, potentially life-threatening! You find yourself standing in the doorway of life, facing some of your deepest fears!

Scripture has numerous stories of very reluctant heroes. When God tapped Jonah on the shoulder and told him to head to Nineveh, he responded by jumping aboard a boat heading in the opposite direction. Gideon resisted God's call to be a mighty warrior by listing all the reasons he was utterly incapable of fighting anyone.

It reminded me of Bilbo Biggin's response, in *The Hobbit*, when he declared, "We are plain quiet folk and have no use for adventures."[58]

There are many reasons that we, like Jonah or Bilbo, may also resist the call. We may be comfortable with our "stuck-ness" in our ordinary life. We may not want the change bad enough to risk it all or we may lack conviction that God deeply cares for us. I have seen so many guys finish the *Conquer Series*,[59] *Sexual Integrity 101*,[60] and *Seven Pillars of Freedom*, and they feel like they have whipped their sexual addiction. Despite this good progress, they still haven't dealt with the issues driving their destructive behaviors. They have checked all the boxes. They have done the work. They have been there, done that, and got the t-shirt—only to experience switching addictions or falling right back into their old patterns a couple of months or years down the road.

> They have missed the fact that God's call on their life has not changed and it will always challenge them to risk it all to help others!

This is precisely the most significant challenge of this book: following Christ in this life is about becoming aware of His call in your soul. There are several reasons why we may not hear it. We may not be ready for it. We may not want it badly enough, or we may not know ourselves well enough to recognize it.

---

[58] J.R.R. Tolkien, *The Hobbit* (New York: Ballantine Books, 1965), 18.

[59] *Conquer Series*, directed by Jeremy Wiles (Stuart: KingdomWorks Studios, 2013), DVD.

[60] Pure Desire Ministries, *Sexual Integrity 101: an 8-week Study for Men, Women, & Churches* (Troutdale: Pure Desire Ministries International, 2020).

The two most important days of your life are the day you were born and the day you find out WHY.

The movie *Braveheart*[61] is the stirring story of William Wallace, a thirteenth century farmer in Scotland, who eventually comes to grips with the WHY of his life. He merely wanted to live in peace, even though the English had killed his father. He sternly rejected the call to make a difference in his world by refusing to fight. Finally, he reached his breaking point when the English magistrate had his wife brutally executed. He finally responded to the call by leading Scotland to rebellion against the brutal king of England.

Mel Gibson's Hollywood rendition of Wallace may not have been accurate in every historical detail. Still, as the Scots faced the overwhelming power of England on the battlefield, his speech was a classic example of passionately expressing the WHY of a man's existence. As Wallace rides his horse back and forth in front of the men with a battle-ready, blue-streaked face, he cries out to the terrified men:[62]

"I am William Wallace. And I see a whole army of my countrymen here in defiance of tyranny. You have come to fight as free men, and free men you are. What will you do with that freedom? Will you fight?"

To which the men respond, "Fight? Against that? NO, we will run; and we will live."

Wallace, turning his horse, confronts the men with the reality of the choices they face: "Aye, fight and you may die. Run and you will live—at least a while. And dying in your bed many years from now, would you be willing to trade all the days from this day to that for one chance, just one chance to come back here and tell our enemies they may take our lives, but they'll never take our freedom!"[63]

When I sat in the theater years ago watching Mel Gibson's speech, I had to wipe away the tears from my eyes. I needed to face the harsh reality that I HAD TO FIGHT for my spiritual freedom on the battlefield of my daily life. At that time, the Holy Spirit was openly challenging me to step aside from my comfortable role of pastoring a large church into an adventure that could cost me everything. I was resisting the change because, as a tenured pastor, I had the system figured out.

God had asked me to give birth to Pure Desire Ministries International and move to potentially ZERO income! My wife and I could lose everything we worked so hard to achieve. I knew exactly how that ragtag group of Scots felt as they faced the certainty of defeat before the power of the English!

---

[61] *Braveheart*, directed by Mel Gibson (Santa Monica: Icon Productions, 1995), film.

[62] *Braveheart*.

[63] *Braveheart*.

It was in the process of risking everything that I profoundly discovered the WHY of my life. I was called to see others set free from what had haunted my life for decades! For all of us, unless we understand the WHY behind not only our recovery, but our whole life, we will continue to resist the call.

You see this challenge in almost every hero movie—the hero's hesitation to respond to the call on his life to change his world. We love to read about David's Mighty Men that we read about in the last chapter. Put yourself in their shoes, however, and it quickly becomes apparent it's an arduous journey. You are saying "yes" to a gargantuan unknown; I mean, how is David ever going to escape Saul's murderous rage? He will not even raise a hand to fight the king![64] They had such courage and conviction for their adventure even in the face of insurmountable odds!

At the other end of the courage spectrum from David's heroes lies the Billy Crystal character in the movie *City Slickers*.[65] It tells the story of a 39-year-old New Yorker by the name of Mitch Robbins. He is tired of his life and his job, and on top of that, his marriage is in trouble. So, he and his two best friends turn in their briefcases for saddlebags and head out to find freedom and adventure in the challenge of learning how to herd cattle at a "dude ranch." Soon they find themselves under the surly leadership of Curley, played by Jack Palance. Curly is an iconic and stoic figure who always seems to have a smoldering cigarette hanging out of the right side of his mouth.

In one scene, Mitch, the city-slicker, is finally facing his fear of Curly as they sit beside a campfire. Curly, as he toys with a very large knife, has told Mitch to put away his annoying harmonica. Mitch's eyes are the size of dinner plates as he watches the blade of Curly's enormous knife reflect the light of the campfire.

Amazingly enough, Mitch apologies for teasing Curly when they first met. He then acknowledges Curly's attempts at scaring him and comments how he is doing a good job of it! Then he faces his fear. Mitch tells him: "If you are going to kill me then get on with it! If not, then shut the hell up! I am on vacation!"[66]

It is a powerful picture of two men learning to respect one another. My favorite scene comes next. The following day, as they are taking care of the herd, Mitch begins to ask Curly a series of personal questions trying to better understand this inscrutable character.

> *Mitch: Ever been married?*
>
> *Curly: Nah!*
>
> *Mitch: Ever been in love?*

---

[64] 1 Samuel 24:6-7 (NIV).

[65] *City Slickers*, directed by Ron Underwood (Beverly Hills: Castle Rock Entertainment, 1991), film.

[66] *City Slickers*.

> *Then Curly begins to share this erotic description of a young lady he saw working in the field one day.*
>
> *To which Mitch excitedly asks: What happened?*
>
> *Curly: I just turned around and rode away.*
>
> *Mitch: Why?*
>
> *Curly: I figured it wasn't going to get any better than that.*
>
> *Mitch: But she could have been the love of your life!*
>
> *Curly: She is…*

At this point, I was thinking Curly sure fits the profile of the classic sex addict I deal with every day in my office: a tough guy who is totally out of touch with his emotions, lives on fantasies, and finds fulfillment primarily in his job. And he is terrified of real intimacy.

Then Curly turns philosophical as he waxes on about the joy of finally bringing the herd to market. He turns toward Mitch, with his ever-present cigarette dangling precariously from the corner of his mouth, and asks a fascinating question.

> *Curly:* **Do you know what the secret of life is?**
>
> *Mitch: No, what?*
>
> *Curly raises one finger and with a twinkle in his eye, he says:* **This!**
>
> *Mitch: Your finger?*
>
> *Curly: Just ONE THING. You stick with that and everything else don't mean sh**!*
>
> *Mitch: That is great but what is the one thing?*
>
> *Curly: That is what you've got to figure out!*

I love the scene where Mitch is left staring at his one raised finger as Curly rides off to help a cow struggling to give birth. This scene is replayed so frequently in my discussion with men who are struggling deeply in their marriage. They are like Mitch: stuck in life or caught in the jaws of another relapse.

Curly's challenge helped me understand a passage of Scripture that had puzzled me for years. In 2 Kings 13:18-19, we find an incident where Elisha challenges the king of Israel to act boldly, illustrating his belief in God's ability to destroy the armies coming against him. When the king only stuck the ground three times, the prophet was angered by his lack of courage. This is what puzzles me: I've read the passage repeatedly and couldn't find any warning to the king of the importance of the moment.

The truth is, he was oblivious to the critical moment because of his fear and his previous choices. The hero's hesitation to God's call on his life may be a normal response, as we have previously pointed out. But to stay frozen in fear is to eventually end up living a life ruled by fear. This is why Elisha declared to the king, "You should have struck the ground five or six times; then you would have defeated Aram and completely destroyed it. But now you will defeat it only three times."[67]

In order to understand Elisha's response to the king, we need to go back to where his story begins and see how he responded to "the call" in his life from his predecessor, the prophet Elijah. The beginning of Elisha's story is rather abrupt but it becomes clear what he considered to be his ONE THING in life.

> *So he (Elijah) departed from there, and found Elisha the son of Shaphat, who was plowing with twelve yoke of oxen before him, and he was with the twelfth. Then Elijah passed by him and threw his mantle on him. And he left the oxen and ran after Elijah, and said, "Please let me kiss my father and my mother, and then I will follow you."*
>
> *And he said to him, "Go back again, for what have I done to you?" So, Elisha turned back from him, and took a yoke of oxen and slaughtered them and boiled their flesh, using the oxen's equipment, and gave it to the people, and they ate. Then he arose and followed Elijah, and became his servant.*
>
> 1 KINGS 19:19-21 (NKJV)

Elijah suddenly interrupted Elisha's life while he was working hard. Elisha was plowing his fields with 12 yoke of oxen, which was not a small farm. He was a hardworking, prosperous man. This is often the way God works in our lives. God has a much bigger agenda than we do and He is not looking for an opening in our schedule.

God will interrupt your schedule and ask you to set aside your plans and bright ideas and follow Him...period!

When has God interrupted your life and suddenly you had to set aside your plans to follow Him?

_____

_____

_____

_____

_____

_____

[67] 2 Kings 13:19 (NIV).

It would be much more convenient if God would give us a year or more to get our life in order and then we would radically follow Him. Truth is, most of us are faced with a "right now" decision with respect to God's calling on our life. The deep double bind we face is the frantic pace of our lives.[68] We want God to move in our lives but we are not ready to move with Him.

If you think it is hard to let go of your failures in the past, then try leaving behind all of your success! I know some of you are saying to yourselves, *I would like to have that problem!* But the truth is, you can be holding on to the wins of the past because you really don't know or trust God to give you any wins in the future.

In my decision to start Pure Desire Ministries, I came to realize I had made my ONE THING the wrong thing! I had built my identity around the growth of my church. Scripture is very clear that God is a jealous lover.[69] He will not allow something or someone else to steal our heart. I will never forget the day I finished preaching my last sermon where I had seen God do so many miraculous things. I walked out the door to starting a brand new ministry, and we had no income, no staff, and didn't have a clue what to do next. But I had finally made the ONE THING the right thing! I had decided to follow the Lord wherever He was leading.

It was through this experience I realized: nothing can hold you back like your past success. Sometimes, it can hold you down more than your failures. And it is important to understand that Elisha wasn't following Elijah because of the hugs and affirmations he would get from his mentor. The Hebrew Prophets were not known for all the warm fuzzy words they would speak, especially Elijah.

"*Go back again, for what have I done to you?*"[70] This is a classic Elijah one-liner. He was essentially declaring to Elisha, "You take care of your past but I am calling you into your future."

Elisha responded to the challenge by taking three steps to deal with his past:

01. He sacrificed the oxen.
02. He used the yokes for firewood.
03. He began to serve Elijah as his servant.

I am sure someone must have made a few comments to him in this process like, "Don't kill the oxen, you will probably need that income down the road!" Or "Don't set those custom made yokes on fire like some cheap firewood! Do you know how much you

---

[68] A double bind is a lose-lose situation we face. The decisions and choices we make are difficult and will cost us something; cost us something to stay the same and cost us something to change. However, one choice will pull us farther into unhealth and isolation. The other choice will lead us toward health and relationships with God and others.

[69] Exodus 34:14 (WYC).

[70] 1 Kings 19:20 (NKJV).

could sell them for on eBay?" But Elisha understood a key aspect to God's way of doing life: **you can't succeed in the things of God if you are counting on some backup plan**.

Elisha decided to follow God's plan for his life and there was no turning back. This is why he could sense what needed to be done in 2 Kings 13. He understood exactly what God was doing and the king didn't have a clue. Elisha had learned the key of going all in and not holding back, while the king was still hedging his bets and playing it safe.

I wonder if there is anything in your life you keep holding on to, and thus, it keeps holding on to you? It could even be your past victories in life. It is something that prevents you from perceiving what God wants to do in your life. Is God saying to you, "Let it go, burn it up! My heart is to move you into a future you can't even conceive of right now!"

> Is there anything you need to let go of because it is keeping you stuck in your life? Or is there a recurring thought or an attitude that keeps setting you up for relapse? What do you need to release from your past failures or victories? Explain.

_____
_____
_____
_____

The willingness of Elisha to sacrifice everything to pursue God's calling in his life resulted in a huge barbecue and blessing for his friends and neighbors.

> Are you living off the sacrifice of others? Or have you realized, there comes a time in life where you need to pay it forward and sacrifice for others? As a result, your life can become a gift to others, especially to your wife and children. Explain.

_____
_____
_____
_____

Elisha knew the profound difference between having something and something having him. This is why he gave up everything so he could step into a future that contained everything only God could give him. **His past successes were not an anchor but an altar** which opened his eyes to see the future the Lord had for him. If your past is your best future, then you are already dead; but you haven't realized it yet!

Probably the most radical part of Elisha's response to God is his decision to become a servant to Elijah. Elisha was a successful man. The text implies he had been a servant to his father for years. He could have so easily said, "Been there, done that, and got the t-shirt!" But he understood the pathway God always takes in the life of a great leader. He moves him up by calling him DOWN. The first step God takes in a great leader's life is to call him to become a more powerful servant.

This is why Curly got it so right and so wrong at the same time!

The Bible gives all of us—single or married—a clear idea of what our ONE THING is all about. In Galatians 5:13, Paul writes, "*You, my brothers…, were called to be free. But do not use your freedom to indulge the sinful nature; rather, serve one another in love.*"[71]

> How are you doing with respect to your calling to serve others in love? What does this look like in your life?

_____
_____
_____
_____

If you are married, a very specific ONE THING God calls you to is found in Paul's declaration of war in Ephesians 5:25-26.[72]

> *And to the husbands, you are to demonstrate love for your wives with the same tender devotion that Christ demonstrated to us, his bride. For he died for us, sacrificing himself to make us holy and pure, cleansing us through the showering of the pure water of the Word of God.*
>
> EPHESIANS 5:25-26 (TPT)

This verse must be seen as the highest call a husband can ever have in his life. And in living out this ONE THING we will find ourselves in hand-to-hand combat with hell. It is unfortunate that most guys I counsel see the warfare as being with their wounded wife. They are resisting the call of God in their lives because their hurting wife's reaction to them triggers their shame and defensiveness. The problem is they will remain stuck in life or caught in an endless cycle of relapse until they stop resisting the ultimate call of God in their life!

---

[71] New International Version (NIV).

[72] We will discover in Stage VII those with the gift of celibacy/singleness and those without the gift are ultimately called to the same love.

How are you doing with respect to your calling as a husband?

    1. Going all out in your love for your wife?

    Where could you improve? (If unsure, ask your wife.)

    2. Giving in the relationship and not taking?

Where could you improve?

3. How do you bring out the best in her through your words and actions?

Where could you improve?

For single guys, in Stage VII we will take an extended look at the focus of the ONE THING that God calls us to.

BE PREPARED TO SHARE WITH YOUR GROUP YOUR ANSWERS TO THE QUESTIONS IN THIS CHAPTER.

In the next stage, we will meet our mentors for the challenging journey ahead. For these chapters, I could think of no one better than my wife, Diane Roberts, to help unpack the importance of our mentors, and ultimately to connect you more deeply to the greatest mentor of all—the Holy Spirit!

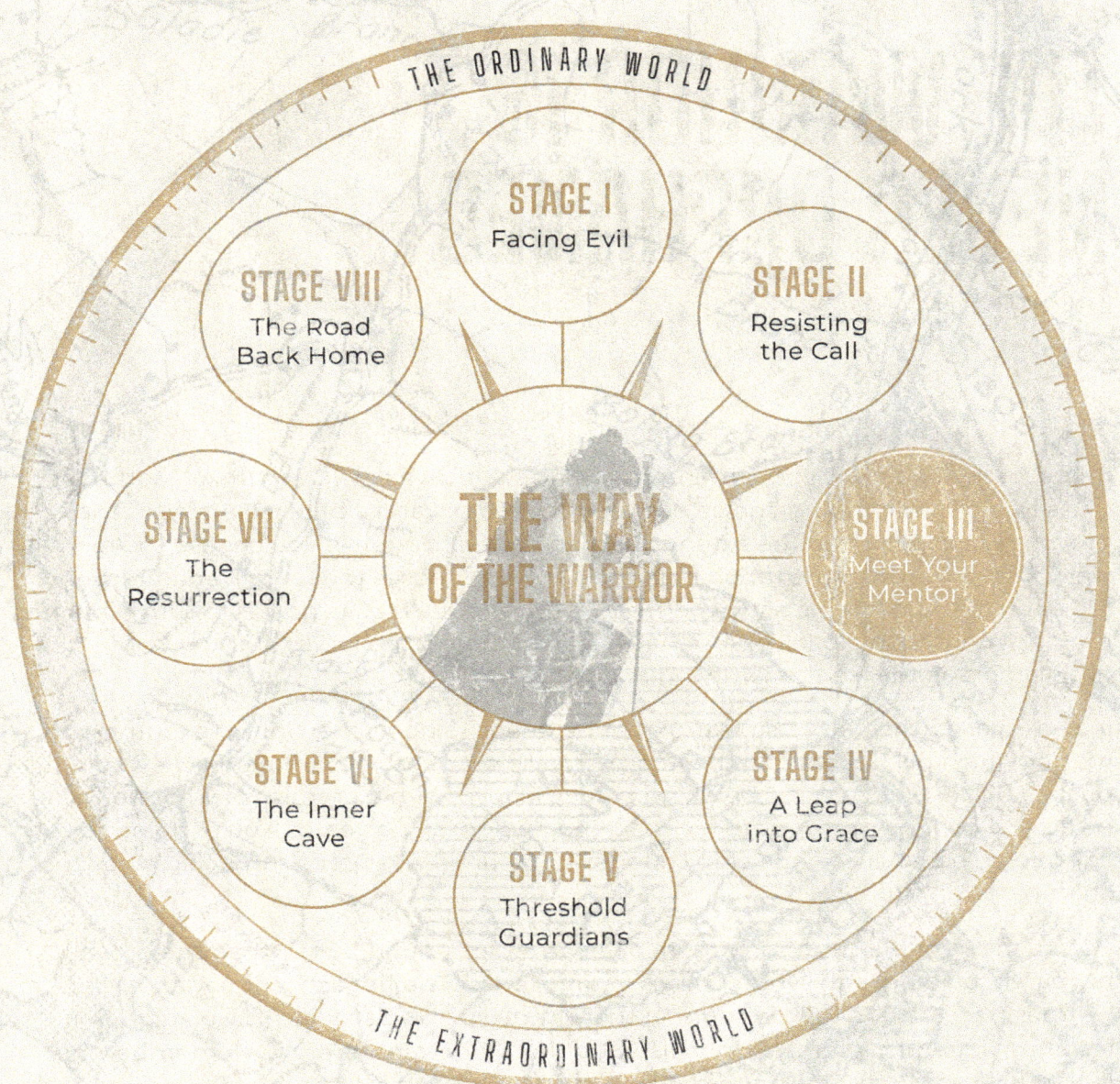

STAGE III
MEET YOUR MENTOR

CHAPTER 5
THE WARRIOR IS NEVER ORPHANED

WITH DIANE ROBERTS

In one of my all-time favorite mentoring movie scenes from *The Matrix*,[73] Morpheus gives Neo a life-changing choice between the red pill and a blue pill. He adds the provocative comment as he extends his hands toward Neo, "If you choose the red pill we will see how deep the rabbit hole goes."[74] Neo chooses the red pill and his eyes are open to the demonic activity of *The Matrix* and realizes its goal is to turn him into nothing more than a pack of AAA batteries. Ultimately the red pills also give him the gift of courage to face the terrifying reality of *The Matrix*.

In some cases, the hero is so fearful that he needs to be pushed into the journey, no matter which pill he takes. In the *Rocky*[75] movie series, boxing trainer Mickey Goldmill pushes *Rocky* Balboa to his breaking point. He gives him a promise of what he will be able to do if he responds to his coaching and doesn't give up: "You're going to eat lightning' and you're gonna crap thunder!"[76] Goldmill was preparing *Rocky* to be a championship fighter.

Few mentors of our time carry more of a pound-for-pound punch than the green, big eared, balding, and syntax-assassinating Yoda.[77] The English language murder he does! Yet, there is such wisdom in the way he speaks because his violation of traditional grammar forces you to listen to the words very carefully. Remember the incident where Yoda challenges Luke to raise his X-wing fighter out of the slime of

---

[73] *The Matrix*, directed by Lana Wachowski and Lilly Wachowski (Burbank: Warner Bros, 1999), film.

[74] *The Matrix*.

[75] *Rocky*, directed by John G. Avildsen (Los Angeles: Chartoff-Winkler Productions, 1976), film.

[76] *Rocky*.

[77] *Star Wars: Episode V - The Empire Strikes Back*, directed by Irvin Kershner (San Rafael: Lucasfilm, 1980), film.

the bog on Dagobah? "Okay," Luke responds to Yoda's challenge, "I'll give it a try."[78] To which Yoda impatiently responds by uttering one of his classic one-liners: "**Do or do not. There is no try.**"[79]

Yoda's response to a young Skywalker has echoed in my heart since the first day I heard it. The violation of grammar makes his words stand apart from the pack of contemporary self-help gurus. Mentors need not be as cryptic or as confrontational as Yoda.

I remember a time I sat in the darkened theater, thankful no one could see the flood of tears streaming down my face. In the movie, *Good Will Hunting*,[80] Will Hunting's counselor, Dr. Sean Maguire, was played exquisitely by Robin Williams. In fact, Williams won an Oscar for his supporting role. His character speaks to the deepest wounds of Will's heart. They both had experienced the sheer terror of being beaten by an alcoholic father. Dr. Maguire lovingly cuts through the tough guy exterior of Will's protective personality and looks deep into his soul as he tenderly declares to him, "It wasn't your fault, it wasn't your fault!"[81] He embraces Will as the tears begin to flow and this is when I lost it as well. I had been raised by a number of abusive stepfathers who were alcoholics and had used me as a punching bag.

Great mentors are invaluable because they often have been where you are, have learned the hard lessons, and can now steer you toward a healing path. They know the haunting questions you may have from traumatic events of your past and they appreciate the obstacles you now face.

Moses speaks these encouraging words to Joshua as he is about to lead the people of Israel into the promised land:

> *"And I commanded Joshua at that time, saying, 'Your eyes have seen all that the LORD your God has done to these two kings; so will the LORD do to all the kingdoms through which you pass. You must not fear them, for the LORD your God Himself fights for you.'"*
>
> DEUTERONOMY 3:21-22 (NKJV)

And, of course, Jesus' words were frequently "mentoring truths" to give the disciples hope in the midst of the challenges they would face.

---

[78] *Star Wars: Episode V - The Empire Strikes Back.*

[79] *Star Wars: Episode V - The Empire Strikes Back.*

[80] *Good Will Hunting*, directed by Gus Van Sant (Los Angeles: Miramax Films, 1997), film.

[81] *Good Will Hunting.*

"These things I have spoken to you, so that in Me you may have peace. In the world you have tribulation, but take courage; I have overcome the world."
JOHN 16:33 (NASB)

These Scripture passages clearly speak to the fact that no one successfully navigates the Hero's Journey on their own.

As we begin this Stage, answer the following questions to get your thinking started.

- Who do you currently look to as a mentor? Who have you looked to in the past?

_____

- If you currently don't have a mentor, how might it benefit you to have a mentor? What steps could you take to find one?

_____

In order to help us understand the role of mentors in our lives, I have asked my wife, Diane Roberts, to take the baton from here on in Stage III.

Ted and I were brought to tears while watching the movie, *I Still Believe*,[82] as the story of singer Jeremy Camp unfolded. Jeremy's love story tells of the highs and lows with his first wife, Melissa, who experienced a miracle of total remission from her cancer during their engagement only to lose her life to cancer shortly after their wedding. Melissa's death was heart-wrenching. At the height of his grief, Jeremy begins asking his dad the WHY questions. "Dad, why after all our prayers was my younger brother born with a disability and not healed? With all your faithfulness to the pastorate, why was your ministry such a struggle? Why would God allow the love of my life to be taken from me?" Jeremy continues in his despair: "I begged God to heal Melissa, what do I do with that?"[83]

---

[82] *I Still Believe*, directed by Andrew Erwin and Jon Erwin (Nashville: Kingdom Story Company, 2020), film.

[83] *I Still Believe*.

Life isn't fair and even warriors on their Hero's Journey often ask WHY as they break through to what God has for them.

> Share some WHY questions you have had with God in your life.

When asked these WHY questions, Jeremy's loving father responded:

"Are Josh's disabilities disappointing? Yes, they are. Did I have big dreams that didn't come true? Sure. Do I understand why Melissa isn't here anymore? No, son and I am sorry. But I do know my life is full. I feel rich and I'm proud of this family. At the time you chose to marry Melissa, to be honest, I didn't agree with you and I didn't understand it. You willingly chose to walk into the fire with her, right beside her all the way to the end. But that is exactly what I do for your mom and you boys. That's what love is and I watched my son do that for his wife. That was a privilege. I don't know the answers to your questions, but I'm proud of you, Son."[84]

Many of us wish we had a father who was there for us, especially in those dark moments, who could speak such wisdom in times of despair.

For many of those who go through Pure Desire groups and/or counseling, there are few who have this kind of dad. In fact, many of the men and women we help have **experienced** abusive or absent dads. Those living with neglect have also **experienced** a lack of attachment whereby their brain was set up to look for addictive behaviors to soothe the pain. These **experiences** shape us! During the first couple of years of childhood when our limbic brain is being developed, we have no way to verbally express our needs. "If our cries were repeatedly met with abuse or neglect, rather than loving care, then we had to learn to self-gratify. Self-gratification is the result of diminished ability to trust others as well as give and receive affection."[85]

Ted was in this situation, having been adopted from birth and raised with seven abusive stepdads. For years, he sought out father figures; but the turning point in his life and in our marriage was his salvation and the filling of the Holy Spirit. Those new spiritual **experiences** began to change his belief system and God began His deep healing work in Ted. One such **experience** came as Ted was reading Romans 8:14-15 (NKJV):

---

[84] *I Still Believe.*

[85] Michael Dye, *The Genesis Process: For Change Groups, Book 1 and 2, Individual Workbook*, 4th ed. (Auburn: Michael Dye, 2012), 174.

*For as many as are led by the Spirit of God, these are sons of God. For you did not receive the spirit of bondage again to fear, but you received the **Spirit of adoption** by whom we cry out, "Abba, Father."*

Shane Pruitt says it this way: "When God saved you, He saved you into a family!"[86]

As Ted read this passage, he saw in his mind's eye a huge pant leg in the corner of the room. (Later Ted jokes that he guessed God's leg was so big He couldn't get both legs in the room). In this vision, he saw himself get up, run over, and cling to the giant pant leg with the new realization that all of us are adopted into God's kingdom. For the first 26 years of Ted's life, he always felt like a misfit being adopted from birth and having seven abusive stepdads. With this new **experience**, something shifted and he knew God would not flake out on him like his previous dads and God would be there for him every step of the way. This was Ted's first personal promise and the beginning of his "father wound" being healed.

Our limbic system can only be changed by new **experience**s because it was originally programmed through experiences.[87] Every hero warrior needs to know God has always been there for him, even if he has felt alone and abandoned.

> What experiences (through pictures, God's words, etc.) have you had with God that reframed traumatic thinking in your life and helped you with a new belief system?

_____
_____
_____
_____

If nothing comes to mind, ask God the Holy Spirit to speak to you as He did to Ted.

Remember, Jesus guaranteed us one important thing on our journey. Right before He faces the Cross, He speaks to His disciples who will soon be launching into their own individual Hero's Journey and says:

*"If you love Me, keep My commandments. And I will pray the Father, and He will give you another Helper that He may abide with you forever—the Spirit of truth whom the world cannot receive, because it neither sees Him nor knows Him; but you know Him, for He dwells with you and will be in you. **I will not leave you***

---

[86] Shane Pruitt Quote, SermonQuotes, January 16, 2019, https://sermonquotes.com/tag/shane-pruitt.

[87] Bessel van der Kolk, *The Body Keeps the Score: Brain, Mind, and Body in the Healing of Trauma* (New York: Penguin Books, 2014), 56.

orphans; *I will come to you...At that day you will know that I am in My Father, and you in Me, and I in you."*

JOHN 14:15-18, 20 (NKJV)

If you had an experience as a child where, even though you may have had parents, you felt alone or like an orphan because of neglect or abuse, passages like this can be part of reframing your experience.

A woman I was counseling had to work through a lot of anger because, as a child, she was sexually abused by her dad. As we worked through all the anger and grieving of her lost childhood innocence she asked, "Diane, where was God? I felt so scared and alone." I replied, "I don't know, let's ask Him." As we prayed, God gave me a picture of Jesus sitting on a front porch swing with His arms wide open. As I shared this picture, the woman began to cry. She said, "We had a front porch swing (which I did not know). I thought it was my safe place because people and traffic passed by the front of our house and I was sure Dad wouldn't hurt me in public. But now I realize it was safe because Jesus was there." This gave her a new **experience** to reframe her traumatic abuse.

> Pick one of the lonely memories you have and ask Jesus where He was for you. Try to picture the memory and let Jesus reveal Himself to you and record what you see.

_____

_____

_____

_____

The power of reframing a wounded experience allows our brain to have a new focus. The woman who was abused no longer has to go back to the memory of the abuse. She has a new picture, underlining the time when she was in her deepest pain, where God was with her on the porch swing. And this has become her new focus.

God saying, "***I will not leave you as orphans,***" emphasizes that He intended for us to walk The Way of the Warrior with the power of the Holy Spirit. It is the Holy Spirit who empowers the warrior.

The Holy Spirit helps the warrior discover his true identity.

If you find yourself replicating the very things you said you would never do, you have probably already discovered trying harder or trying not to be like Mom, Dad, (you fill in the blank) _____ never works.

Rather than trying **not** to be someone they were hurt by, the warrior needs to discover who God has called him to be. Mentors have the capacity to see something in the hero that the hero cannot see in themselves. Often, it takes a mentor to help you discover who God has called you to be.

We will talk about the many mentors Ted and I have invited into our lives over the years in the next chapter; but the most powerful mentor of all, hands down, has been the Holy Spirit, especially when I found myself stuck in behaviors I tried to change on my own.

I remember vowing I would never be like my mom and grandma who were both very critical, negative, and judgmental. I didn't even see I was perpetuating these traits until I saw them displayed in my eight-year-old daughter. At first, I was in denial and thought that negative, critical spirit had skipped a generation! The Holy Spirit rolled up His sleeves and began mentoring me through my denial and showed me step-by-step how to change my unwanted behavior.

Although, at the time, I didn't know how it started, I realized I was dealing with a generational curse passed down through three generations. When the enemy sees an opening of unwanted and/or sinful behavior, Scripture tells us we can give Satan access or strongholds in our lives.[88] Scripture also says these strongholds or curses can go to the third and fourth generation. I knew a generational curse needed to be renounced, so I asked my daughter if she would pray this prayer with me:

> *Dear Lord,*
>
> *We ask your forgiveness for walking in negative, critical, and judgmental behavior. We take responsibility for those behaviors but we also realize this was passed down to us through the generations. Therefore, we bind whatever spirits think they have access or a right to harass and influence us and we renounce their existence in our lives. We ask that you, Holy Spirit, would fill us afresh with your spirit of love, in Jesus name, Amen.*

I then asked my daughter to hold me accountable if she saw any of this old nature and she gave me permission to do the same for her. We knew there were habit patterns we needed to change. And guess what? It worked! For a month. Then I saw some of these habits creeping back in. Now what?

I told the Lord we were trying hard not to be critical, negative, and judgmental. This is when I heard Him say, "**Diane, I don't give you power NOT to be something. I give you the power to become who I have called you to be.**" In amazement at this revelation, I asked, "God, who have you called me to be?" He took me to Galatians 5:22, where the Fruit of the Spirit is listed. The word kindness jumped out at me.

---

[88] Ephesians 6:12.

This is when I heard Him say, "I have called you and your daughter to be gracious." I laughed and reminded the Lord I had never seen this lived out growing up; how could I possibly become a gracious woman of God? In my spirit I sensed God saying: "Surrender to My Spirit, and ask Him to help you become a gracious woman of God; and He will teach you."

Sure enough, because I yielded to Him, thereafter when I came to a fork in the road and my flesh would normally respond in the old patterns, I would hear a whisper from the Holy Spirit, sometimes just a little nudge, and He would show me how to replace the old patterns with graciousness. God the Holy Spirit was teaching me to walk in the Spirit (graciousness) rather than in the flesh (a critical, negative, judgmental spirit).

I love how brain science is validating a lot of what the Holy Spirit does in our lives. If you are familiar with the Baader-Meinhof Phenomenon you understand what I am referring to.[89] If this is new to you, think of it this way: after purchasing a new car, all of a sudden, you see that model and color of the car everywhere. Ted and I were recently on a walk and I noticed there were a number of white cars on our 1.5-mile walk. We started counting them and discovered there were over 60 white cars! Either our conscious awareness was more dialed in or white cars miraculously were popping up everywhere. **The point is, you can't understand something you are not aware of; but once you see it, you can more easily change it.** This is what the Holy Spirit was speaking personally to me. It's as if He said, "Diane, you are a gracious woman of God and now your new focus will give way to new actions."

List an unwanted behavior you have been stuck in and have tried hard "not" to do.

I challenge you to look at the summary list of Galatians 5:22-23 and find the Fruit of the Spirit which would be the opposite of the unwanted behavior you have unsuccessfully tried to change. Chances are, the enemy has tried to wound you in your gifting of who God has called you to be.

---

[89] Baader-Meinhof Phenomenon, Dictionary.com, June 28, 2022, https://www.dictionary.com/e/tech-science/baader-meinhof-phenomenon/.

Circle the Fruit of the Spirit and the opposite behavior you have tried to stop.

FRUIT OF THE SPIRIT	OPPOSITE ATTITUDES AND BEHAVIORS
Love	Unforgiveness, anger, bitterness, judgmental
Joy (Gladness)	Depression, heaviness, loneliness, isolation
Peace/Patience	Easily irritated, frustrated, perfectionistic
Kindness/Goodness	Negative, critical, judgmental
Faithfulness	Inability to trust, lack of commitment, procrastination
Gentleness	Rude, harsh, aggressive

As we identify the Fruit of the Spirit we want help in living out, it can be useful to repeat this beautiful, short prayer: "Lord, help me understand what you had in mind when you made the original me."[90]

In light of this prayer, who do you think God is saying you are?

_____
_____
_____
_____
_____

If you are not sure, ask God to show you. Then pray a prayer yielding and asking the Holy Spirit to lead you and to mentor you in how to walk in the Spirit rather than the old fleshly ways. The enemy can counterfeit the Gifts of the Spirit but he has none of the Fruit of the Spirit. Satan has no peace, patients, kindness, gentleness, or self-control. The Fruit of the Spirit is the evidence of the great work God wants to do in each of us.

Over the years, I have marveled at how many have commented on either myself or my daughter's graciousness; I have had to chuckle and say, *Thank you, Lord. Your Holy Spirit was the mentor who led us and guided us.*

Recently, Ted and I had the privilege of visiting my daughter's daughter. I was taken aback by her sharing a conversation she had with her college professor who had

---

[90] Joanna Weaver, *Having a Mary Spirit: Allowing God to Change Us From the Inside Out* (Colorado Springs: Waterbrook Press, 2006), 234.

made a harsh decision to throw her out of her college class because she had gone to visit her parents during Covid-19. My granddaughter, although feeling hurt because she didn't know about the consequences ahead of time, graciously responded to her professor by saying, "I can't imagine how hard it is for you to work during covid—having to break the one class I am taking into six separate classes to accommodate social distancing. I am thankful you value this program enough that you are going the extra mile to provide this class."

Upon new information the professor received about the school allowing a football team from another county to live in the dorms at the school and practice football, she came back to my granddaughter and said she was thankful for a student who so graciously recognized her hard work. The professor also said, "I have decided I can't throw a paying student out of my class while football players from another county are allowed to use our campus." With my granddaughter's gracious words and the revelation of the school's decision about the sports team, God came through on her behalf.

Generational curses are real. But the Bible says the blessings are greater than the curse and go to a thousand generations.[91] I witnessed the power of the blessing of graciousness to the next generation in my granddaughter through this experience.

Jesus says something amazing about the role of the Holy Spirit as our mentor. He asked his disciples to follow Him and, later in John 14:12, he said something astounding: "...*he who believes in Me, the works that I do he will do also; and greater works than these he will do, because I go to My Father.*"[92]

How could this be possible? The works Christ did included healing the sick, casting out demons, miracles, words of wisdom and knowledge—even raising the dead! Remember in Philippians 2:6-7, Scripture states that Jesus limited (emptied) himself while He was on earth. Every miracle Jesus did was through the **power of the Holy Spirit**. In Acts 1, Jesus tells the disciples to wait in Jerusalem to receive the power of the Holy Spirit—the same power Jesus used to do the miracles He did.

The disciples were born again in John 20:22 when Jesus breathed on them and said receive the Holy Spirit. But it was in Acts 2, the Holy Spirit fell on the disciples who were waiting in Jerusalem as Jesus directed and they were filled with the Holy Spirit. Throughout the book of Acts, we see the disciples doing the same miracles Jesus did after being filled with the Holy Spirit.

The great news is the power of the Holy Spirit is still available today. Peter declared in Acts 2:38 that this power was available to those he was speaking to and their children and all the generations to come. The Holy Spirit is the greatest mentor. Have you asked Jesus to fill you with the Holy Spirit?

---

[91] Deuteronomy 5:9-10 (NIV).

[92] New King James Version (NKJV).

Maybe in my sharing about my daughter and granddaughter and hearing how the Holy Spirit has worked in our lives, you might be asking, "How could that be?" Ted and I had been born again but we realized we were lacking in power, especially the healing and transformative power talked about throughout the Gospels and the book of Acts. We wanted more. We wanted, as the disciples on the day of Pentecost, to be filled with the Holy Spirit. As we sought the Holy Spirit earnestly, His power began to fill our lives in new ways.

This same power is available to you. You may have asked Jesus into your heart but if you have never asked to be filled with the Holy Spirit and you realize you need more power to walk with Jesus, I encourage you to pray this simple prayer and believe God will honor it as He did with the disciples, and as He did with Ted and me.

> *Dear Lord,*
>
> *I thank you Jesus for salvation and that You died for me. Thank you for forgiving my sins. Thank you also that You, Jesus, went to the Father so You could send the Holy Spirit. I know when I said "yes" to Jesus, I received the Holy Spirit and now I am yielding myself to be cleansed, empowered, and filled with the Holy Spirit. I yield myself to the cleansing of my heart and the gifts you want to flow through me for helping others. Have all of me, Holy Spirit, and fill me with your life and power. In Jesus name, Amen.*

If you prayed this prayer, ask the Holy Spirit to now be your mentor and look to Him to lead you into a new adventure in the Spirit, with new power to walk in the Fruit of the Spirit.

> Pray your own prayer and ask Him to mentor you in how to walk in the Fruit of the Spirit you circled in the previous exercise. Answer the following questions to process the work of the Holy Spirit more deeply.

> What could you do to give the Holy Spirit more room to be your mentor?

_____
_____
_____
_____
_____
_____
_____
_____

Who is someone you trust and respect that you feel is led by the Holy Spirit? How could you learn from them?

What fears or reservations do you have about being mentored by the Holy Spirit?

NOTE: We know that theological traditions differ on the method or timing of how the Holy Spirit fills us. What we can all agree on from the New Testament is the clear reality of the Holy Spirit with us. No matter your faith tradition, we hope this chapter helps you focus on embracing the Holy Spirit to be your mentor in a powerful way.

BE PREPARED TO SHARE WITH YOUR GROUP YOUR ANSWERS TO THE QUESTIONS IN THIS CHAPTER.

CHAPTER 6
THE MENTORED WARRIOR BECOMES THE MENTOR

BY DIANE ROBERTS

In the last chapter, we talked about the importance of the Holy Spirit mentoring us. This is a vital role God has in our recovery. But our recovery—even being mentored—cannot be confined to God alone! Because we are wounded in community, it is important to be healed in community. This means within the Body of Christ. Every Hero's Journey has mentors.

Ted mentioned the significance of these in the Introduction: Mentors appear in our lives "in preparation for the transition from the ordinary to the extraordinary. They are often heroes who have survived life's trials and are now passing on the gift of their knowledge and wisdom."

As a review, we have already seen a number of mentor types:

- Obi-Wan Kenobi gives Luke Skywalker his father's lightsaber and a new understanding of the Force.
- Morpheus gives Neo a pill that helps him see how deep the rabbit hole goes.
- Mickey Goldmill pushes *Rocky* Balboa to become a champion.

Here are a couple more:

- John Keat (played by Robin Williams), who was the teacher in *Dead Poets Society*,[93] challenges his students with "carpe diem"—seize the day and make your lives extraordinary. John Keat confronts his students with their mundane routine of academia and calls them to embark on a new adventure.
- Dorothy, in *The Wizard of Oz*,[94] learns incredible lessons from everyone she encounters as she journeys through the land of Oz, especially from her three fellow travelers: a man of straw, a man of tin, and a talking lion. They become allies and mentors who teach her lessons about the brain, the heart, and courage.

---

[93] *Dead Poets Society*, directed by Peter Weir (Burbank: Touchstone Pictures, 1989), film.

[94] *The Wizard of Oz*, directed by Victor Fleming (Beverly Hills: Metro-Goldwyn-Mayer [MGM], 1939), film.

Share how any of these characters remind you of mentors in your past. Who has challenged you to embark on a new adventure? Explain.

_____
_____
_____
_____
_____

In your opinion, what qualities does a good mentor possess?

_____
_____
_____
_____
_____

Who has helped you get unstuck from your past wounds or the relapses that keep recurring? Explain what they did and how it helped.

_____
_____
_____
_____
_____

Maybe, like many of us, you have not had a John Keats figure in your life; but all of us have had people who knowingly or unknowingly poured positive attributes into us to help us become the person we are today.

In our healing journey, we often think about the negative contributors who inflicted trauma and pain which has stunted our emotional growth. In fact, growing up, some of our negative thinking and debilitating self-talk may have come from those closest to us. But for a moment, let's look at the flip side and appreciate the positive attributes we were taught, even by some of those who may have also wounded us.

In the chart that follows, identify mentors who have added positively to your life.[95] I have included the Holy Spirit because I realized when I did this exercise, many attributes were communicated to me by God through the Holy Spirit working in my life. You may want to add teachers, coaches, or others in the extra column provided.

DAD	MOM	SPOUSE	HOLY SPIRIT	GRANDPARENTS	OTHERS

On the chart, assign the following positive attributes to those who have poured into your life.

- ☐ adaptable
- ☐ adventurous
- ☐ appreciating
- ☐ artistic
- ☐ athletic
- ☐ bold
- ☐ cheerful
- ☐ Christian
- ☐ compassionate
- ☐ confident
- ☐ content
- ☐ courageous
- ☐ creative
- ☐ dependable
- ☐ discerning
- ☐ disciplined
- ☐ energetic
- ☐ enthusiastic
- ☐ faithful
- ☐ financially-blessed
- ☐ forgiving
- ☐ fun-loving
- ☐ generous
- ☐ gentle
- ☐ giving
- ☐ God-fearing
- ☐ good listener
- ☐ good provider
- ☐ gracious
- ☐ hardworking
- ☐ healthy
- ☐ honest
- ☐ hopeful
- ☐ hospitable
- ☐ humble
- ☐ insightful
- ☐ integrity
- ☐ inventive
- ☐ joyful
- ☐ kind
- ☐ leader
- ☐ loving
- ☐ loyal
- ☐ musical
- ☐ nurturing
- ☐ obedience
- ☐ optimistic
- ☐ organized/detailed
- ☐ patient
- ☐ peaceful
- ☐ persevering
- ☐ playful
- ☐ productive
- ☐ prosperous
- ☐ respectful
- ☐ responsible
- ☐ safe
- ☐ self-controlled
- ☐ sincere
- ☐ stable
- ☐ teachable
- ☐ thankful
- ☐ thoughtful
- ☐ trustworthy

---

[95] Michael Dye, *The Genesis Process: For Change Groups, Book 1 and 2, Individual Workbook*, 4th ed. (Auburn: Michael Dye, 2012), 184-185.

What did you learn from this exercise? What attributes did you find coming to mind most frequently? Why do you think this is?

_____
_____
_____
_____
_____
_____
_____

Anthony Tjan, CEO of Boston venture capital firm and author of **Good People**, says:

> The best mentors can help us define and express our inner calling, but rarely can one person give you everything you need to grow.[96]

Over the years, Ted and I have tried to balance our lives with three types of mentors:

Type One

Someone who could pour into our lives because of their skills and/or their ability to walk in the Spirit and follow Christ closely. This is typically someone who is ahead of us in life, age, or responsibilities. They are guiding us to walk on paths they have already traversed.

FOR DIANE:

As a young Marine wife, I looked to women who understood the military and could help me adjust to moving to different duty stations and deployments. The greatest advice I remember getting from one wise woman was, "I always try to find something I like in every new duty station we are assigned."

In my first year of teaching, I spent time with the other fifth grade teacher, Mrs. Green, working on lesson plans that she had spent years fine tuning.

---

[96] Julia Fawal, *The 5 types of mentors you need in your life*, Ideas.TED.Com, https://ideas.ted.com/the-5-types-of-mentors-you-need-in-your-life/#:~:text=%E2%80%9CThe%20best%20mentors%20can%20help,everything%20you%20need%20to%20grow.%E2%80%9D.

In a season where I longed to pray more, I spent hours praying with an intercessor, Dorcas, who had grown up in an intercessory church.

As a pastor's wife, I will never forget the best advice I ever received. I was beginning to resent feeling like I was in a "fishbowl" and the senior pastor's wife, Devi, said, "Diane, do you resent being a mom?" I immediately said, "No, I love being a mom." Her response was, "Look at your pastor's role as being a mom to your entire church family." Her words freed me and changed my whole perspective.

FOR TED:

I naturally looked for mentors in the military, especially in the flying game. There was a major who literally took me under his wing. This was very unusual for a major to pour into the life of a second lieutenant! It just wasn't done; flight instructors treated lieutenants like a form of "low life" who basically didn't deserve any attention at all. But Major Burns, for some reason, took a liking to me and spoke of my unique abilities.

Pastor Butch Plumber mentored me in how to love the flock. He would hold people at the altar and weep with them. I was able to walk out and preach love, acceptance, and forgiveness for the next 24 years as a pastor because of Pastor Butch.

> Of the mentors you've considered so far, who is someone who has poured into your life and what wisdom have you gained from this person?

_____
_____
_____
_____

Type Two

A peer or wingman, someone who is walking the journey with us and we are able to pour into each other's lives. A peer mentor is on our level and easy to relate to since we are sharing in the journey together.

FOR DIANE:

I have been part of the Pure Desire clinical team for the past few years and have gleaned so much from other counselors. With these fellow counselors, it has been a give and take relationship that helps me fine tune my counseling skills.

FOR TED:

Tyler Chinchen is someone who has been there for me as the Pure Desire clinical team was formed. He has become someone who not only has been there in every tough decision I've made in the development of the team, but he was the perfect person to lead the team once I had to take on the personal and difficult battle with Parkinson's disease.

Of course, no one has ever been a peer and co-pilot mentor like my wife. She has loved me and believed in me despite the crazy and angry man I became once I returned from Vietnam. I was literally out of my mind for two years. Through her incredible love for me, I came face-to-face with the scandalous love of God. Pure Desire Ministries became what it is today simply because I was outrageously loved by Diane!

> Share one or two examples of those who are or have worked with you in your life. These are what I call **"iron sharpens iron"** relationships.[97] (It may include members of your Pure Desire group and/or your wife):

If it was difficult for you to fill in the previous list, realize this is what God has in store for you. If you are married, it might start with your wife.

Part of mentoring others is seeing what they cannot see about themselves and speaking it into their lives. Ted has always seen me as being more gifted and capable than I have seen myself. I can attest to the fact that there is a big footprint in the middle of my back side; where he has believed in me and pushed me into areas I would not have gone without his coaxing and encouragement. In our church, I built a large women's ministry and a healing ministry for our entire church. Ted also encouraged me to get trained in helping women who have been betrayed because of their spouse's secret sexual behavior. I also started a group for women struggling with sexual/love addiction. The curriculum I wrote has been foundational for women who go through Pure Desire today. This would not have happened without a loving husband who had great confidence in me.

---

[97] Proverbs 27:17.

What are some gifts you see in your wife? How could you encourage and support her in the greater development of these gifts?

___

Most of the men we counsel have recognized the power of having their wife pour into their lives. Clinical analysis has shown that the willingness of husbands to accept their wife's influence predicted marital success 80% of the time.[98]

One of the most powerful and difficult gifts a husband can receive from his wife is her Emotional Impact Letter that she presents during the clinical disclosure process. She helps him see his blind spots and how his addictive behavior has impacted her life. Part of the Hero's Journey is for the husband to face his wife's pain without moving into a place of shaming himself. This was true for one counselee who received an Emotional Impact Letter. Here is an excerpt from his wife's letter:

> *I gave you the benefit of the doubt when I got that anonymous email outing you. I believed you, wholeheartedly, when you told me you were faithful and that you would never cheat on me, that you would tell me if you were ever tempted to so that I could have the chance to work on our marriage with you. I have been standing by you through the worst possible garbage that a marriage can be hit with. I have gone a step beyond that to attempt to reach out to you when I feel like I have been ripped to shreds with my self-esteem in*

___

[98] John M. Gottman and Nan Silver, *The Seven Principles for Making Marriage Work* (New York: Harmony Books, 1999), 121ff.

the toilet. Because I care for you. Because I love you. But no. I am your father... your abuser. No one is in your corner. You talk a lot about people not being in your corner, and maybe that was true in the abuse you suffered as a child. But you have, in turn, become the perpetrator of the very thing you hate.

You have never been in my corner, not for one day of our relationship. From the get-go you were lying and cheating, getting your fix from pornography and gratuitous sex with other women, all the while stringing along a fairytale romance with the one that you "loved." Would you call that being in my corner? I was always alone in this. I was alone when I married you and took those vows; the only one taking them in sincerity. I was alone when I was pregnant and gave birth to our three beautiful children while you continued in your addictive behaviors. I was alone in every heart-to-heart conversation, every trip, every memory we ever made. I was alone. And now, here I am after all that you've done. Still here. If not for certain about reconciliation, at least certain about the fact that I want to see you healed, that I believe you are worth loving.

Her courageous letter, with her raw honesty, opened her hero husband's heart to face his own sin, guilt, and trauma in an amazing way. This hero was able to receive influence from his wife, taking full responsibility for his betrayal and not only wrote his wife a Restitution Letter, but took it to another level by writing to her parents, owning his sin, apologizing for the hurt he caused their daughter, and asking for their forgiveness. Here is an excerpt from the letter he wrote and gave to her parents:

Firstly, I am so sorry for how I have hurt you both. I lied to the both of you, hiding my sexual addiction, and shattering your daughter's world, your granddaughters' worlds, because of my lies, my deceits, and my deceptions. I broke all the vows that I made to my wife, filled my head with such horrors, gave my body away to such filth, and was that filth also. I endangered my family through my selfish and awful actions, and those actions will echo for some time. I was completely unfaithful to your daughter, cheating on her so many times, with so many different women, and watching so much pornography. I lied to her and to you about what kind of man I was.

This man's words to his in-laws shows how much he had opened his heart to his wife and allowed her words, and her honesty, to mentor and mature him! Because this husband and wife *both* chose to do the hard work for healing, within a year of going through counseling and groups, their relationship was powerfully restored to the point where they are now helping others who are struggling in Pure Desire groups.

NOTE: *The Emotional Impact Letter and the Letter of Restitution are powerful aspects of the Pure Desire counseling process. For more information on taking this journey for yourself, please contact the counseling office at info@puredesire.org.*

Type Three

A reverse mentor would include those I was pouring into, usually someone younger. And despite their age, they were oftentimes able to give me much needed feedback and a fresh perspective from their experiences and different generational views. Here are some examples:

FOR DIANE:

In our church's healing ministry, I would often glean amazing insights from those who were being healed. One woman who had endured tremendous sexual shame from her father, I was able to help her work through a lot of her trauma. At the end of our work in processing her memories, the Lord told her to do two things. First, find a large red cloth and wrap yourself in it. As she did, she heard her heavenly Father say, "I have covered you with my blood which has cleansed you of all the shame from your past." Then the Lord directed her to cover herself in a white cloth and as she did the Lord said, "My blood has cleansed you from your shame and trauma and you are now as white as snow." This was a graphic illustration of God's healing in her life which also spoke volumes to me about God's incredible love for hurting women!

FOR TED:

After leading Pure Desire groups for over 30 years, one of the things I so love is seeing young men rise up to join the fight. I have developed the habit of looking for a young man I could really pour my life into and I would ask them to co-lead the group with me. Without exception, all had a deep father wound in their soul and, as I watched them experience healing, I gained new insights in how my heavenly Father was healing me. In the process, I came to understand how deeply Father God loved me!

> Realize, your mentoring words to others can be life-changing.

In my early years of teaching, Chris was one of my students in a Christian school for kindergartners. He was a hellion in every way. If there was a fight on the playground, Chris was the instigator. In the classroom, he was mean and would purposely pull a chair out from under his classmates. Chris's mother was a fellow teacher in the school, so I spent a lot of time on my knees praying for him, trying to understand why he was in my classroom.

Three months into the school year we put together a Christmas program for parents in the form of a mime. The children reenacted a modern-day version of the Good Samaritan. The story started with a little boy coming home from a baseball game and some bullies jumped him, beat him up, and stole his baseball bat and glove. Two people, including the pastor's daughter, ignored him as they passed by his bleeding body. Finally, a boy who was delivering newspapers from his wagon stopped, helped him into his wagon, and found help for him.

As I was giving out parts, I asked, "Who wants to be one of the bullies?" Chris immediately raised his hand and my first thought was he would be perfectly cast for the part and wouldn't even need to act! As I was about to appoint him head bully, God spoke to me and said, "He is supposed to be the Good Samaritan." I knew it must be God because I would have never pictured Chris in this light. In fact, it took some convincing to get Chris to agree to this until I mentioned he would be the only one pulling the wagon.

Miracle of miracles: after many rehearsals, at the end of our Christmas program where Chris was pulling the wounded boy in his wagon—the curtains were closing, the parents were applauding—and something began to change in Chris's heart. He was still all boy, but I believe this was the beginning of him seeing himself differently. Seeing himself the way God saw him, as a Good Samaritan. This experience helped teach me to never underestimate what God can do in someone's life.

> When has someone you are mentoring, a younger sibling or even one of your children, caused you to have a new perspective? Explain.

_____
_____
_____
_____
_____
_____
_____
_____

It may be within your healing journey where you will be able to help someone have new understanding or perspective. **It is through helping others that you truly grow as a warrior in the Hero's Journey God has designed for you.**

Back to the previous story, one of the reasons our hero husband grew so much and saw so much restoration was his decision to not only share with his wife and her parents but also share with his three daughters.

Here is an excerpt from a letter to his oldest daughter who was only eight at the time. Notice how he is able to communicate in an age-appropriate manner and also cover his wife so his daughter will realize the pain her mom was enduring:

This is going to be a very difficult letter, because while you are the smartest little girl I know, this is a very hard thing to say to you.

You know why mom and I had to separate last year. It was because I lied to mom, many, many times. Our whole marriage, actually. What I lied about is even harder to tell you. You see, when I married mom, I promised that I would love her, only want her, and only be with her. Well, that's what I lied about. Not the loving mom part–that is true.

I know this past year has been very hard on you and your sisters, with all of you having to go from house to house on weekends, not knowing what was going on. I am so sorry for that; I wish we didn't have to do that. Now you know why mom had to ask me to leave and why we had to live apart for more than a year: your mom needed to know that I could change, that I wanted to change, that I wanted her, and you, back too.

So I started getting help: going to groups, getting counseling, going to counseling with mom to help her heal from all the lies I told her.

I love you so much, and I am working to be the daddy that you deserve and need. You need me to be strong, to be honest, to be loyal, and even when I'm afraid, to tell the truth. I am going to be the daddy that you need, the daddy God saw that I could be, and is helping me become.

I love you.

Daddy.

This dad realized his words, his honesty, and his amends to his daughter could change the next generation.

I have often wondered if David in the Bible could have done more to change his children's decisions. In Acts 13:36, we read of David, who appears in the Hall of Fame as a biblical hero in Hebrews chapter 11, "*...after he had served his own generation by the will of God, fell asleep...*" But look at what happened in the history of the next generation. His son Absalom tried to kill David and did kill his brother Amnon for raping his sister.[99] Did David honestly share with his children his adultery with Bathsheba and his scheme to have Uriah killed?[100] Would some of the pain his children went through have been mitigated if David had these honest, vulnerable, hard conversations with each of them?

---

[99] 2 Samuel 15-19 and 2 Samuel 13:23-38, respectively.

[100] 2 Samuel 11.

Deuteronomy 5:9-10 says, "...I, the LORD your God, am a jealous God, punishing the children for the sin of the parents to the third and fourth generation of those who hate me, but showing love to a thousand generations of those who love me and keep my commandments." Notice how the blessing's influence is FAR more powerful than the curse! But every hero must decide if he will mentor the next generation so blessings will flow.

Imperfect warriors realize generational changes only happen when there is honesty and truth is shared with their children. When the next generation can make sense of what they have experienced, only then is change possible in their lives. Warriors also know this type of intentional mentoring conversations have to be ongoing as their children grow, if generational change is to take place.

Now let's put all of this together. As you have thought about mentors these last few lessons, who is God putting on your heart for this next season of your journey?

Who could mentor you and pour into your life—a wise sage or guide?

Who could be your wingman or peer mentor?

Who could be a reverse mentor—someone younger or following you?

What steps can you take to spend more intentional time with the three people you have listed?

How might God be asking you to change the next generation?

What would this change require on your part?

It has now been over 40 years since I was Chris's teacher. I don't know how his life played out, but when I get to heaven I am going to ask Chris, "How did God use you as a Good Samaritan?" I am confident that God used our relationship to shape his life, even as it shaped mine!

Lord, thank You that You can use us as mentors and healed healers. This is the ultimate purpose of our Hero's Journey.

Based on what you've learned so far, how is it helping you become a Compassionate Warrior? Be specific in your answer.

BE PREPARED TO SHARE WITH YOUR GROUP YOUR ANSWERS TO THE QUESTIONS IN THIS CHAPTER.

INTERLUDE
BEFORE YOU READ ANY FARTHER… A WARNING AND A BLESSING.

A WARNING: The remainder of this book should begin to radically change your life! This is why I have posted this warning. Change can never occur in life until we understand what we are actually struggling with and can answer this question: What is causing me to stay stuck in my faith?

I have already mentioned how the title of this book may be a real head-shaker for you: *The Compassionate Warrior*. It sounds as if the ultimate paradox somehow ended up as a title. In a sense, this is true and I make no apologies for the title. The greatest biblical truths are typically described as a paradox. For example, could you please explain to me the Trinity? Or how Christ was fully human yet, at the same time, entirely God? Or the clash of the two concepts: the sovereignty of God and the free will of man?

You can't explain these three concepts through human logic, yet they lay at the heart of what we believed to be true concerning God's character. I find the modern church's amnesia and aversion totally puzzling concerning one of God's most fundamental qualities: He is a warrior.

> *The Lord is a warrior; the Lord is his name.*
> EXODUS 15:3 (NIV)

> *The Lord will march forth like a mighty hero; he will come out like a warrior, full of fury. He will shout his battle cry and crush all his enemies.*
> ISAIAH 42:13 (NLT)

Every man wants to make a difference in this hurting world. Man was created in the image of God, who He himself is the great warrior. Thus, God gave you a warrior's heart because you were created in His image and you were born into a world at war. But to be a warrior also means that we will face opposition. Have you realized your life is opposed? Your love is opposed. Your hopes, your dreams, your joy are all fiercely opposed by hell. The amount of hardship you will endure in this life is determined by the depth of your warrior's heart. In as much as it's up to him, a man in a difficult marriage can hang in there once he discovers the warrior inside. The heart of a warrior says to hell, "I will put myself on the line for my wife. I will not allow the enemy to have his way!"

And a warrior knows it is a waste of time to ask, "Why is life so hard at times?" Instead, he takes this hardness as the call to battle, to rise and face the challenge, and sets his "face like flint" as Jesus did in fulfilling his life's calling.[101]

Therefore, I need to warn you, from this point on the following chapters will probably really challenge you. You will turn the page and find yourself facing some issues you may have avoided for years!

While most people just want to survive, a warrior wants to thrive. They want to stand atop the defeated carcass of the enemy, like David did, and lift worship to God! It isn't about being rescued from a rough day. It's about breaking through into what God has for them. Warriors love to make the enemy feel the sting of sweet revenge. They live by a unique formula: **the favor God has on their lives, plus pressure, leads to payback!** Warriors have the tenacity to hold on to the Lord even when everyone else fades away.

A BLESSING: a prophetic promise for your days ahead.

I hear God speaking over your future and the plans he has for you saying, "My Son, in this next season in your life, I am going to radically deepen your perspective. You will begin to understand both the power that is in you and the power that stands behind you.

I will cause you to occupy a higher place in My affection. And a higher place of sensitivity in the Spirit is awaiting you. The places in your life where you have been counted out will become the places of your greatest encounters with me.

The enemy will reveal to you and others where the hand of God is upon you. For this purpose, I have allowed the enemy to rise up so that I may demonstrate My power over you, IN YOU!

Fear is always present in the fight, otherwise there wouldn't be a struggle. When you live above fear, however, it becomes a weapon in your hand; and you will take it, you will drive it into the heart of the enemy! This is my prophetic promise to you!"

---

[101] Isaiah 50:7 (NIV).

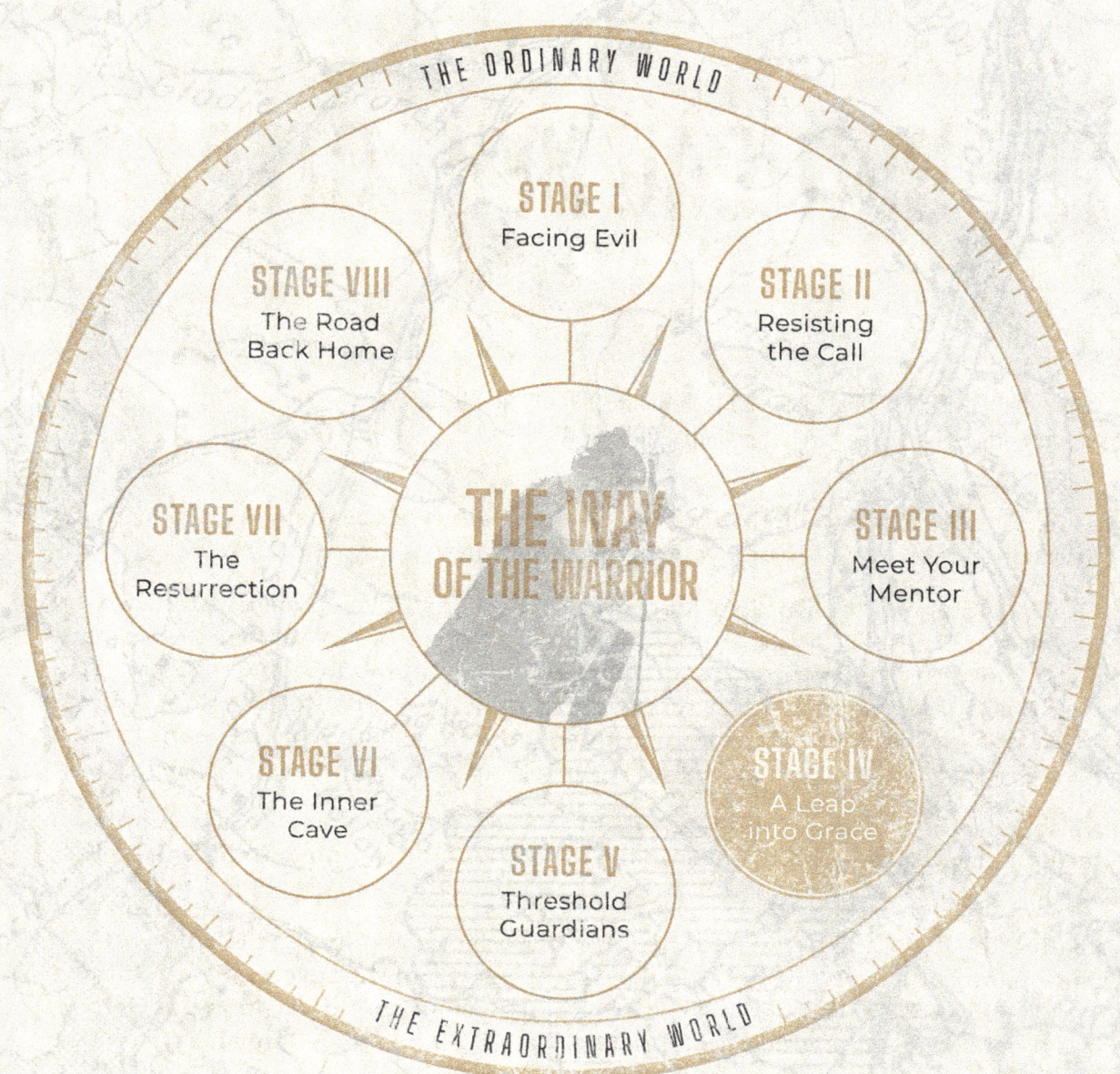

STAGE IV
A RADICAL LIFE-ALTERING LEAP INTO GRACE

CHAPTER 7
THE CRITICAL NEXT STEP

> ❝ Our purpose is the reason we take the leap in the first place. Our passion is the torch that lights our leap.[102]

In life, purpose is not found in what we do but in *why* we do what we do. If you can figure out the *why* in life, then you can deal with almost any *what* or *how*.

It is at this stage of the warrior's journey that the Christ-follower takes a radically deeper step. The leap of faith entails moving from the ordinary to the extraordinary in life. The hero crosses the threshold into the supernatural. Joseph Campbell's leap of faith is faith in the process of the Hero's Journey. As a Christ-follower, our faith is the person of Christ, not a process. In this stage, we will learn what it means to trust deeply in Him to transform us. For our champion is ALIVE; He is not dead!

We serve a Warrior King. Therefore, one of the best places to be with Him is on a battlefield, outnumbered by the enemy, as you hear Him laugh in their face and say, "Is that all you've got?"

Hearing the joy of the battle and the heart of God for you is incredible! Spiritual warfare is all about discovering the majesty of Jesus and the sovereignty of God the Father. Our sense of wonder in God's sovereignty is our confidence and our victory. This perspective kills passivity and enables us to act while the enemy is still raging.

Despite the enemy's antics, our hearts can remain at rest. I am convinced, our intimacy with God can become the most intimidating weapon we can have against our enemy. I am looking forward to the time where I can walk in such confidence and rest in Christ to the point where I confuse and exhaust the enemy. He will end up pulling out his hair in frustration because his attacks only make me stronger in Christ. If he ignores us, we will rip him apart. If he openly attacks, the Lion of the tribe of Judah will devour him. Victory is inescapable. We cannot screw it up for God because God has already won in Christ. He can do something majestic and sovereign in any moment; and our joy is to find out what He is up to.

---

[102] Will Craig, *Living the Hero's Journey: Exploring Your Role in the Action-Adventure of a Lifetime* (Greenville: Live and Learn Publishing, 2017).

God, our loving heavenly Father, is always peeling away what we see as defeat and revealing His grace. He is not obsessed with our sin—He has dealt with it by fully judging it in Jesus. We have always been forgiven. We must learn to revel in it! We must come to the place where we fully forgive ourselves as well. It is critical that we come to the place of realizing our heavenly Father is not disillusioned with us, for He has never harbored any illusions about us.

Now the tricky part in all of this is our great God will send us out into battle facing overwhelming odds with absolutely ridiculous battle plans. "Here is what I want you to do. March around the enemy's position for seven days and then shout," He will say, winking at you the whole time.[103] It sounds like a bunch of lambs being sent out to the slaughter. Fortunately, we may be lambs but we have the mighty Lion of Judah as our friend. We are not sent out defenseless but as warriors who are vulnerable to who He is. When we are truly vulnerable to God, the Lion will always walk with the lamb.

There is a scene from *The Wizard of Oz*[104] where I laughed out loud the first time I saw the old classic. The Tin Man, Cowardly Lion, and Scarecrow are attempting to rescue Dorothy from the Wicked Witch of the West's castle. They are facing impossible odds! There are countless legions of well-armed soldiers guarding the castle. They came up with a plan that sounds just like God. Here is the plan: commandeer some uniforms and weapons and march straight into the castle, like you own the place. I cracked up when they marched into the castle with the Cowardly Lion's tail sticking out the back of his uniform and his knees knocking so loud you could hear them. I thought, "What a picture of myself at times!"

When I first arrived at the church I pastored for over 20 years, I discovered the finances were a total mess. They were 4.5 million dollars in debt beyond the building payment and only a couple hundred people in attendance. There was absolutely no way we could make it! Yet, the Lord spoke to my heart that He would clear away the debt in one year. So many times as I stood up to speak each weekend, my knees were knocking just like the Cowardly Lion's. Yet somehow I knew the Lion of Judah was walking with me. He paid off the debt in one year to the exact day—and this was despite the fact my knees were knocking the whole time!

What impossible dreams has God placed in your heart?

---

[103] Joshua 6:2-17.

[104] *The Wizard of Oz*, directed by Victor Fleming (Beverly Hills: Metro-Goldwyn-Mayer [MGM], 1939), film.

What do these dreams say about your God-given purpose?

What leap of faith do you need to take to experience God's extraordinary grace in your life's purpose?

In Stage II, we looked at the Old Testament prophet Elisha and his interaction with the King of Israel. I want to revisit this story as it has another application to this stage of our journey as well. This is a marvelous story depicting one who trusted God but was held back—the King of Israel—and because of this, received so much less than he could have received from the Lord. In stark contrast, the other man—Elisha—held nothing back, he went for it! As a result, he received a stunning blessing from God. In fact, his boldness is perceived by some as a bit off-the-page but he was just a man totally surrendered to God.

> *Now Elisha had been suffering from the illness from which he died. Jehoash king of Israel went down to see him and wept over him. "My father! My father!" he cried. "The chariots and horsemen of Israel!"*
>
> *Elisha said, "Get a bow and some arrows," and he did so. "Take the bow in your hands," he said to the king of Israel. When he had taken it, Elisha put his hands on the king's hands.*
>
> *"Open the east window," he said, and he opened it. "Shoot!" Elisha said, and he shot. "The Lord's arrow of victory, the arrow of victory over Aram!" Elisha declared. "You will completely destroy the Arameans at Aphek."*

Then he said, "Take the arrows," and the king took them. Elisha told him, "Strike the ground." He struck it three times and stopped. 19 The man of God was angry with him and said, "You should have struck the ground five or six times; then you would have defeated Aram and completely destroyed it. But now you will defeat it only three times."

2 KINGS 13:14-19 (NIV)

First of all, Elisha directs the king to shoot an arrow out of the east window. This was the direction from which the actual enemy was approaching. Next, he asks Jehoash to strike the ground with his arrows and then becomes irritated because he only struck the ground three times instead of six. I can picture the king saying to Elisha, "It would have been helpful to know that little detail, that I needed to strike the ground six times instead of three."

Have you ever felt like you are missing something because you are not experiencing all that you know God has for you? That is the excruciating agony of relapse. It is striking the situation that stands against us once, twice, three times but nothing happens and so you quit.

Elisha was upset because the king stopped before he gave everything he had. He stopped before he had used his last arrow! Relapse is living stuck in the space between the third and the sixth arrow. Where we give God what we think He wants but not everything we have. The king was holding on to some of his arrows for another time.

Make a quick list of the "arrows" you are letting go of (or you feel God is asking you to let go of) through this journey.

Example: Arrow 1: My need to always be right.

- Arrow 1: _____
- Arrow 2: _____
- Arrow 3: _____
- Arrow 4: _____
- Arrow 5: _____
- Arrow 6: _____

Now to understand Elisha, you have to go back in the story to 2 Kings 2 when he was in a critical transition in his life. This was a time in his life where he was following a man with whom he knew God was with…Elijah.

> *When the Lord was about to take Elijah up to heaven in a whirlwind, Elijah and Elisha were on their way from Gilgal. Elijah said to Elisha, "Stay here; the Lord has sent me to Bethel."*
>
> *But Elisha said, "As surely as the Lord lives and as you live, I will not leave you." So they went down to Bethel.*
>
> *The company of the prophets at Bethel came out to Elisha and asked, "Do you know that the Lord is going to take your master from you today?"*
>
> *"Yes, I know," Elisha replied, "so be quiet."*
>
> 2 KINGS 2:1-3 (NIV)

I love Elisha's response. He is a prophet with an attitude and an edge! The story continues with Elisha refusing to leave Elijah's side as he travels to Jericho and eventually to the banks of the Jordan river. Then the story becomes absolutely fascinating.

> *Elijah took his cloak, rolled it up and struck the water with it. The water divided to the right and to the left and the two of them crossed over on dry ground.*
>
> *When they had crossed, Elijah said to Elisha, "Tell me, what can I do for you before I am taken from you? "Let me inherit a double portion of your spirit," Elisha replied.*
>
> *"You have asked a difficult thing," Elijah said, "yet if you see me when I am taken from you, it will be yours—otherwise, it will not."*
>
> *As they were walking along and talking together, suddenly a chariot of fire and horses of fire appeared and separated the two of them, and Elijah went up to heaven in a whirlwind. Elisha saw this and cried out, "My father! My father! The chariots and horsemen of Israel!" And Elisha saw him no more. Then he took hold of his garment and tore it in two.*
>
> *Elisha then picked up Elijah's cloak that had fallen from him and went back and stood on the bank of the Jordan. He took the cloak that had fallen from Elijah and struck the water with it. "Where now is the Lord, the God of Elijah?" he asked. When he struck the water, it divided to the right and to the left, and he crossed over.*
>
> 2 KINGS 2:8-14 (NIV)

"What can I do for you?" This is the question you hear when you refuse to stay where you are and, instead, decide to give everything to God. I think this is the question you don't get asked until you refuse to stay behind.

"I'm going where you are," Elisha told Elijah, "because where you are is where God is!" **These kinds of folks don't tap out in life.** This is a place, however, where few folks have the courage to go.

Elisha's response to the question, "Tell me, what can I do for you…?" is simply stunning! Have you ever seen someone whose life was a legend and thought to yourself, "If I could have half of what they have experienced, if I could have half of their success, that would be incredible!" Have you ever thought this? Not Elisha. He said, "I don't want half, I want double! I don't want this life because I have lived this life. Now I know what God can do. I want a double portion of your life!" Yet this is not an arrogant request because in Hebrew culture Elisha was essentially asking Elijah to treat him as his firstborn son. He is so bold that he is asking to take the family line to new heights in obedience to God! And Elijah's response to him, "You have asked a difficult thing…" is emphatically declaring that this is something only God can do.

Did you notice that Elisha cries out the same words the king did but with a totally different meaning. Elisha was not crying out in despair but declaring that the Lord is more powerful than death. He realized what an incredible mentor Elijah had been to him but he was seeking God, not just Elijah. When he struck the waters of the Jordan he was asking for something BIG! He was asking, "God, are you still with me, and if so, show me your power!"

What are you asking God for in your life?

Once you let go of what you have been holding on to define yourself, a gracious God will always ask, "What do you want Me to do for you?" This is the starting point of our radical leap into God's grace! It can be a tough question to hear in the midst of a difficult transition, especially in a time when there is upheaval in your life. A time when all the things you saw as permanent are now falling apart. You can respond in two ways: either seeing it as a crisis, or you can realize God is setting you up to let go of the past so you can receive your future.

Ultimately, you realize that it would be a tragedy if one day you saw all the things you longed for in life, the things you hungered for in your soul, the dreams of your heart never came to pass. And why? You wouldn't let go of what you had. You never asked BIG enough! You never received all that God had for you.

When I surrendered my life to Christ, I didn't know any better but to ask God for BIG things. I started praying for my fellow pilots and I prayed BIG. As a result, 50% of the students I instructed came to Christ and 30% of the flight instructors did as well. It was like seeing a brothel converted!

Then in seminary, I was told that it was selfish to pray for God to use you. Instead, you were to pray for God to use others. I understand they were trying to protect us from pride, but I eventually came to believe that this is a very faulty view of faith in our God who answers BIG prayers. I cannot control how much God acts in someone else's life. **But I am responsible for how much I let my passion for God grow in my life.** Here is the great part: if God gave us everything we passionately wanted to do, to help others, it would never run out. He would never say to the guy standing behind me in line, "I am sorry. But apparently, God just ran out of blessings. Ted drained God of all His blessings." **The truth is, God never runs out of blessings for those who hold nothing back.**

No wonder Elisha was upset with the king. He looked at the king who was willing to strike the ground only three times and stopped. Elisha refused to ask for less; instead, he asked for more. He was the kind of man, if God told him to strike the ground, he would have hit the ground with everything he had. **You cannot receive everything God has for you until you lay down everything you have and ask God for more.**

The cycle of relapse in your life will never stop until your passion for sexual health and for God's purposes in your life becomes far stronger than the power of the addiction. And this whole process starts, after the painful process of letting go, by asking God for BIG THINGS to help others. One thing I have learned through the years is that addicts do not realize just how big our God is...certainly much bigger than their addiction. If you do not feel forgiven, truly forgiven, then you cannot have the power God has for you.

Yes, we are weak and broken and not deserving, but we have a God to whom that doesn't matter. He wants us, but He wants all of us.

> In the space below, rewrite the arrows/the things you need to let go of in your life. Things that you may love or things you are holding on to in case God doesn't come through for you. These arrows are usually built around your deepest fears in life.

> As you lay down each arrow, what BIG request from God comes to mind? Where do you want God to use you to touch the lives of others? Spend some significant time in prayer and thoughtfully answer the following questions.

EXAMPLES:

Arrow #1: *My need to always be right.*

My BIG request from God: That He would make me the most empathetic person in my wife's life. That I would be quick to listen and slow to speak.

Arrow #2: *My need to always protect myself when we get into an argument.*

My BIG request from God: That He would make me much more patient, by helping me face my fears. That I would learn to hear my wife's heart instead of just reacting to her words.

Arrow #1: _____

My BIG request from God:

_____
_____

Arrow #2: _____

My BIG request from God:

_____
_____

Arrow #3: _____

My BIG request from God:

_____
_____

Arrow #4: _____

My BIG request from God:

_____
_____

Arrow #5: _____

My BIG request from God:

_____

Arrow #6: _____

My BIG request from God:

_____

BE PREPARED TO SHARE WITH YOUR GROUP YOUR ANSWERS TO THE QUESTIONS IN THIS CHAPTER.

CHAPTER 8
TRICKY JAKE—PART 1

As we have walked through our arrows in life and chosen to trust God with our future, the next part of this stage on the Hero's Journey requires us to make a radical, life-altering leap into grace. We must be willing to leave what we know behind us and step boldly into the supernatural realm of God's control.

This isn't easy to do, but it's possible when we understand two dimensions of grace. **The first dimension of grace is this: when we get what we don't deserve from God.** In other words, we can't earn God's grace because He gives it to us freely. We will look at this kind of grace here in Chapter 8 and then cover the second dimension of grace in Chapter 9.

Far too many churches have failed to connect effectively with hurting people in today's world. If the church you attend does this well, praise God! But many churches have basically taken the same approach in proclaiming the gospel as one more challenge to "do better." Try harder! Be more committed! Stop sinning! Be good!

But instead of screaming at us "DO BETTER!" like a frustrated drill sergeant, grace whispers to us, "I want to do this for you." And instead of persuading us with the typical challenge, "Come on, try harder," grace gently says to us, "I have done the hard work for you. Rest in Me and My power at work within you. And never forget: I love you no matter what."

A friend recently made a very interesting analysis of many Christians he knew, as to why they looked so miserable: "They are suffering from a hardening of the 'oughteries.' They never feel like they have done enough in life to get God's blessing. They are constantly telling themselves they 'ought' to have done more. And this is why they feel so miserable!" It's true—many Christians are trapped in the insanity of trying to be good enough to earn God's blessing. They haven't realized the power of Romans 1:17 which is called a gateway verse by many theologians.

> *For in the gospel the righteousness of God is revealed—a righteousness that is by faith from first to last, just as it is written: "The righteous will live by **faith**."*
> ROMANS 1:17 (NIV)

This single verse set Martin Luther and John Wesley free to leap into God's grace. Wesley returned to England after experiencing a total failure as a missionary to the Native Americans. He wrote in his journal of his spiritual condition at the time while crossing the Atlantic: "I went to America, to convert the Indians; but oh! who shall convert me?"[105] God powerfully answered his question as a friend read Martin Luther's comments concerning Romans 1:17. Wesley noted, "I felt my heart strangely warmed" as he listened to Luther's comments about the verse.[106]

Where have you struggled with feeling you have not done enough in your life to deserve God's blessing?

Now I am not much of a Broadway musical kind of guy, but a number of years ago my wife and daughter-in-law talked me into experiencing *Les Miserables*.[107] I use the word "experiencing" because I didn't see a musical; **I experienced it.** Like no other movie or theatrical production I have ever been to, it opened my eyes to an understanding of grace and a renewed hunger for heaven while I struggled to deal with the challenge of living in a painful world. The title can be loosely translated as "the miserable ones." The musical is not your typical Broadway drama but is a bitter prayer of agony which ends in a final wedding scene that makes a follower of Christ and their heavenly reward almost palpable.

As I sat there, I was totally blindsided by the power of the musical. I held back the tears with everything I had until I heard the words of the song, *Empty Chairs at Empty Tables*.[108]

> **There's a grief that can't be spoken,**
> **There's a pain goes on and on.**
> *Empty chairs at empty tables,*
> *Now my friends are dead and gone.*
> *Here they talked of revolution,*
> *Here it was they lit the flame,*

---

[105] John Wesley, *Journal of John Wesley* (Chicago: Moody Press, 1951), 53.

[106] John Wesley, *Journal of John Wesley*, 64.

[107] *Les Misérables*, directed by Tom Hooper (Universal City: Universal Pictures, 2012), film.

[108] Eddie Redmayne, "Empty Chairs at Empty Tables." Track 36 on *Les Misérables: The Motion Picture Soundtrack Deluxe*. Universal Music Group, 2013, CD.

> *Here they sang about tomorrow*
> *And tomorrow never came.*
> ***...That I live and you are gone...***

As those words impacted my soul, I began to sob out loud. That very day, I was striving to understand why I was alive and a lot of guys I knew never came back from Vietnam. Or if they did come home, they were physically or mentally never the same. The only answer I could come to was the same one the hero of the musical, Jean Valjean, came to—GRACE!

In Valjean's Soliloquy song, we hear and feel the pain of his life.[109]

> *My life was a war that could never be won*
> *They gave me a number and murdered Valjean*
> *When they chained me and left me for dead*
> *Just for stealing a mouthful of bread...*

(Then he tries to understand the actions of the bishop who protected him from being arrested again.)

> *...He gave me his trust*
> *He called me brother*
> *My life he claims for God above*
> *Can such things be?*

Now why is it so hard for us to come to grips with God's grace in our lives? The answer: every man I have ever helped break free from their sexual struggles, at some point in their past, they were given a label on the "Name Tag" of their life and have been chained to it ever since! Therefore, their natural tendency was to try and get the label off their soul by deserving God's favor. But once they understand that grace can only be received, it is never earned, this is when the relapses stopped. Once they experience GRACE, they finally understand that their life was claimed by God.

If others could see the unconscious Name Tag you wear on your heart, the names or labels others projected on you, what would they see? These names are deep, limbic beliefs we are often not consciously aware of until something triggers us.

For example, when you experience conflict with your spouse or in another close relationship, what are some of the names you immediately put on yourself? (*e.g., loser, not good enough, defective, doesn't measure up, tries hard but isn't smart enough, or intelligent but never gets things done.*)

---

[109] Hugh Jackman, "Valjean's Soliloquy." Track 3 on *Les Misérables: The Motion Picture Soundtrack Deluxe*. Universal Music Group, 2013, CD.

Fill in your name tag.

HELLO
MY NAME IS

These Name Tags we wear unconsciously on our hearts can have a huge impact on our daily lives because upward of 80% of the decisions we make come from our subconscious brain.[110] The Scriptures refer to this part of your brain as your heart. The heart or limbic system is foundationally programmed by around age six.[111] Therefore, your family of origin gives you the basic or default window through which you perceive your world; and this perspective operates totally outside of your conscious awareness. This is why Scripture tells us to invite Jesus into our hearts not just into our brain or mind.

When we are born again, what happens? Our spirit is made alive, our prefrontal cortex[112] or higher reasoning center of our brain receives life transforming information through Scripture reading and sermons, but our limbic system must be reprogrammed!

If you are ever going to get the right Name Tag on your heart then you must truly come to **EXPERIENCE** your prophetic or personal promises. Your limbic system is only reprogrammed through positive new experiences which directly address the limbic lies planted there usually from your family of origin. The limbic system is not programmed simply with new data or information.

Our limbic responses are often tied to past painful experiences. If we respond in anger, we puff up to control the situation. If we shut down, we shrink back and choose to isolate. Both of these options are limbic. The only way to face these difficult moments, to be present and stand our sacred ground, is to rehearse our promises.

---

[110] Daniel J. Sielgel, *Pocket Guide to Interpersonal Neurobiology: An Integrative Handbook of the Mind* (New York: W.W. Norton & Company, 2012), 1-5, 13.

[111] Linda Graham, *Bouncing Back: Rewiring Your Brain for Maximum Resilience and Well-Being* (Navato: New World Library, 2013), 202-210.

[112] Bessel van der Kolk, *The Body Keeps the Score: Brain, Mind, and Body in the Healing of Trauma* (New York: Penguin Books, 2014), 60-65.

When have you responded "limbically" in your marriage or to someone close to you?

_____
_____
_____
_____

What personal promise has God given you to combat this limbic response?

_____
_____
_____
_____

In the Old Testament, you meet an individual who had "second best" on the Name Tag of his life from the beginning. In the book of Genesis, Jacob is the second-born son of Isaac. Jacob, or "Tricky Jake" as I like to call him, is the riverboat gambler of the Old Testament. He learned to deal from the bottom of the deck at an early age. Apparently, Jacob never got over the fact that his older brother beat him in the race down the birth canal. Esau won the race and showed up big, red, and hairy. Looking like a red baby Chewbacca,[113] he was named Esau which means "hairy." The second-place finisher showed up grasping the heel of his older brother and was named Jacob which means "holder of the heel" or "supplanter." Esau grew up as a rough and tumble outdoorsman. He was daddy's favorite son, whereas Jacob was a momma's boy.

But here is the critical fact I don't want you to miss: the boys grew up in a family where, at any given moment, at least one of their parents didn't think they were good enough! Parents can either propel their kids to pursue God's plan for their life or train them to react and posture in life. Name Tags that are placed on your heart don't just affect you in your childhood, they can impact you as an adult as well.

In Genesis 27, we find Tricky Jake pulling a con on his nearly blind dad to steal his brother's blessing as the firstborn son. I used to feel sorry for Jacob because Scripture tells us it was his mom who came up with the scheme and he got blamed for it.[114] But once I realized Jacob was likely 76 years old at the time, it seemed inappropriate for him to blame all of his problems on poor potty training! He had learned to posture and scheme his way through life to get what he wanted but **God couldn't bless who he pretended to be!**

---

[113] Chewbacca is a fictional Wookiee warrior in the *Star Wars* franchise, created by George Lucas.

[114] Genesis 27:6-10.

Once Esau discovered how Jacob had conned his dad and stole his birthright, he had only one goal in life—to annihilate Jacob! So, Jacob ran for his life and God loved him enough to allow him to run to a man named Laban and his household. He ended up spending the next 21 years of his life trying to outmaneuver and outwit Laban who was the king of the cons. Jacob learned the hard way that, sooner or later, the trickster will be tricked and the player will be played. Until he came to the end of himself, he couldn't come to the beginning of God's deep work in his life. Jacob was headed into a wrestling match he could never win. A wrestling match with God!

After spending more than 30 years helping men find freedom, I have learned that sometimes hitting a brick wall in life can be a blessing in disguise. I remember one pastor who was leading a huge church and had just been appointed to his dream job of leadership. The problem was, he had been living a secret life for years and it was starting to catch up with him. It soon became public knowledge that he had an affair at a previous church. This is when the dream became a nightmare! In one week, he lost everything—his coveted pastorate, his reputation, and it looked like his wife and daughters were finished with him as well. I had only been counseling with him for several weeks when his life blew apart. At the time, his pain had reached an insane level; he couldn't medicate it away and could no longer run from it.

Like Jean Valjean, his life had become a war that could never be won. In an absolute rage, he screamed at me through the phone, "I am going to kill you and then I will kill myself!" I know this was a horrible response from a clinical perspective, but I sensed the Holy Spirit provoking me to challenge him as a man of God. I smiled, then began to laugh out loud and said to him, "Could you please reverse the order on those actions?"

As you might have expected, this infuriated him even more and he only yelled louder, "Why are you laughing?" I gently spoke to him saying, "Congratulations, you have reached rock bottom. Now God can do the miraculous in your life!"

He later confided in me, "That was the turning point in my healing."

In Genesis 32, we find the turning point in Jacob's life:

> *He took them [his wives and children] and sent them to the other side of the river with all that he had. Then Jacob was left alone. And a man fought with him until morning. When the man saw that he was not winning he touched the joint of Jacob's thigh. And Jacob's thigh was put out of joint while he fought with him. The man said, "Let me go. For the morning has come." But Jacob said, "I will not let you go unless you pray that good will come to me." The man asked him, "What is your name?" He said, "Jacob." And the man said, "Your name will no longer be Jacob, but Israel. For you have fought with God and with men, and have won."*
>
> GENESIS 32:23-28 (NLT)

Jacob, like my pastor friend, found himself alone and lost everything he had been scheming so hard to obtain. When asked, "What is your name?" I'm sure Jacob must have thought to himself, *That is a silly question to be asking me after you broke my hip!*

A number of scholars identify the strange individual who Jacob wrestled with as a person identified as a man yet, at the same time, called God—being a pre-incarnate appearance of Christ. And Jesus doesn't ask us silly questions.

If you remember, 21 years prior to this wrestling match, Jacob was asked the same question by his blind father as he was about to steal his older brother's birthright. His father asked, "Who are you?" and he answered with a lie, "I am Esau."[115] This time he spoke the truth: "I am Jacob, the deceiver, the heel grabber, the broken one!"

Notice how Christ responded to Jacob's honesty about himself and the fact he would never let go of God. In verse 28, God declared to Jacob, *"Your name will no longer be Jacob, but Israel. For you have fought with God and with men, and have won."*

It is so important for us to understand exactly what God was saying to Jacob. Most guys hear God saying to a man who struggles, "Tired of being who you are? Want to be someone different? Shazam! Your wish is granted!" This is not biblical grace. Instead, this is what Dietrich Bonhoeffer called cheap grace.

"Cheap grace is the preaching forgiveness without requiring repentance, baptism without church discipline, Communion without confession, absolution without personal confession. Cheap grace is grace without discipleship, grace without the cross, grace without Jesus Christ, living and incarnate."[116]

You may be thinking, *Wait a minute! This sounds like religious performance; like trying harder, which you have said will never lead to freedom, especially when we are struggling with something as deep as sexual addiction.*

But Dietrich deeply understood the character of God and His grace.

For example, when God encountered Moses in the burning bush and Moses asked His name, He didn't just respond with the puzzling statement, *"I AM WHO I AM."*[117] He also expressed His character in the startling description, *"I am...the God of Abraham, the God Isaac, and the God of Jacob."*[118]

God was declaring for all of human history in identifying Himself with Jacob as well as Israel:

> ▸ I am the God of your mistakes.

---

[115] Genesis 27:18-19.

[116] Dietrich Bonhoeffer, *The Cost of Discipleship* (New York: Touchstone, 1995), 45.

[117] Exodus 3:14.

[118] Exodus 3:6 (NASB).

- I am the God of all the parts of you that you don't want anyone to see. (Which is the source of most of the lies we tell as we struggle with our addiction.)
- I am the God of your struggles as well as your victories.

It is fascinating to note that Jacob is called by both names throughout the rest of the Bible. Why? Change is never easy and, therefore, it is important for you to be as gracious with yourself as God is gracious with you. Discovering who you are and who God has called you to be is a **lifelong journey**.

> Where do you have a hard time being gracious toward yourself? Where does the Holy Spirit need to help you in experiencing God's grace toward yourself so you can be more gracious toward others?

> Instead of viewing yourself through the Name Tag you listed earlier, what NEW NAME do you think God has for you? What is your true identity, by His grace?

MY NAME IS

The grace of God is our strength and hope which we see so clearly in the life of Dietrich Bonhoeffer. He was a pastor in the midst of World War II in Germany. He found the strength to confront the cruel insanity of Hitler's Nazi regime which resulted in his execution while most of the church of Germany kept silent.

After witnessing Bonhoeffer's execution, a Flossenburg doctor reported, "In the almost fifty years that I have worked as a doctor, I have hardly ever seen a man die so entirely submissive to the will of God."[119] Dietrich was a man who understood the grace of God and was able to stand his sacred ground in the face of terrifying opposition, even as he battled with his own weakness and doubts. **He was truly a Compassionate Warrior!**

> BE PREPARED TO SHARE WITH YOUR GROUP YOUR ANSWERS TO THE QUESTIONS IN THIS CHAPTER.

---

[119] Eric Metaxas, *Bonhoeffer: Pastor, Martyr, Prophet, Spy* (Nashville: Nelson Books, 2020), 464.

CHAPTER 9
TRICKY JAKE—PART 2

One of the greatest questions I have ever been asked came from a Navy flight instructor who showed up at a Bible study I was leading early on when I came to Christ. This Navy pilot had experienced a rare malfunction in the launch sequence off an aircraft carrier that had resulted in him ejecting into the sea. As a result, the 90,000 ton carrier ran right over the top of him. Miraculously, to everyone's surprise, he survived, and except for a damaged eardrum, in one piece!

Because of this experience, he looked directly at me in the midst of the other pilots attending this Bible study, and asked a huge question: "I believe in God," he declared emphatically, "but who the hell is this Jesus Christ?"

I exploded in laughter; I had never heard anyone express this question in such a manner. His experience of grace—only God could have brought him through this event—had opened his heart to faith in a new way! I had just seen a vivid example of the second aspect of God's grace in our lives. Grace means that God not only gives us what we don't deserve, **but God's grace also provides us with the ability to change**.

Understanding this is so important because if you don't realize this truth, you are saved by grace but spending the rest of your life trying to change by your efforts. Once you grab hold of this truth and stop trying to get free by working harder through your efforts, this is when you will finally break the cycle of relapse.

There is a passage in Luke 2 that so shocked me, I initially thought there must have been a misprint or mistranslation. But after carefully checking the Greek text, the New International Version translation was "spot on."

> *And the child grew and became strong; he was filled with wisdom, and the grace of God was on him.*
>
> LUKE 2:40 (NIV)

The Passion Translation, a more recent rendering of the passage, deeply grasps the theological truth of the text.

> *The child grew more powerful in grace, for he was being filled with wisdom, and the favor of God was upon him.*
>
> LUKE 2:40 (TPT)

The astonishing truth proclaimed in Luke 2:40 is that the grace of God enabled Jesus **to become who he was meant to be**. He was fully God, but he was also fully man, and as fully man, grace enabled him to grow, become strong, and filled with wisdom! Therefore, there is absolutely no way any of us are ever going to become all Father God has called us to be apart from God's grace. If Jesus needed to grow more powerful in grace, I am sure we are going to need to do precisely the same thing!

Where do you need to grow in experiencing the grace of God in your life?

_____
_____
_____
_____

What has prevented you from leaning into and trusting God in your life?

_____
_____
_____
_____

Where in your life have you tried to change by your own efforts? What helped you finally realize it wasn't working?

_____
_____
_____
_____

After leading guys through *Seven Pillars of Freedom* for the past ten years, one of the things I found deeply frustrating is how many of them struggled to understand the truths revealed about their Arousal Template in Pillar Five. Now I am not the quickest bear in the woods, so it took awhile for God to help me realize why the guys in my groups were struggling. My hope was they would start looking at their sexual fantasies and listening to their lust. Sexual fantasies are the highway signs located on the well-traveled pathway of our past wounds. They also help us understand the current mental mountains blocking our path to freedom. The fact I had missed was that **apart from coming to an understanding of God's grace, the shame in their lives would keep their heads down and they would continue to drive into one mental mountain after another**!

In childhood, many of us have experienced neglect, relational craziness, isolation, pain mixed with sexual arousal, or outright sexual abuse, and these formed the foundational programming for our limbic system. This programming sets us up to repeat these experiences in our unwanted sexual behaviors as adults. This is why we will find ourselves "doing stupid again!" The pattern is so deep, we can't just forget what happened in our past and "get on with life." These past experiences trigger our limbic system and overpower our prefrontal cortex. We end up living in Romans 7:18-19 again!

> *But I need something more! For if I know the law but still can't keep it, and if the power of sin within me keeps sabotaging my best intentions, I obviously need help! I realize that I don't have what it takes. I can will it, but I can't do it. I decide to do good, but I don't really do it; I decide not to do bad, but then I do it anyway. My decisions, such as they are, don't result in actions. Something has gone wrong deep within me and gets the better of me every time.*
>
> ROMANS 7:18-19 (MSG)

My point is that our sexual struggles don't just randomly appear in our lives. The sexual conflicts and fantasies are there for a reason. If we want to stop the insane cycle of relapse, if we want to find freedom, it always begins with identifying our woundedness expressed in our sexual fantasies and conflicts!

In counseling, as a man lists his destructive sexual behaviors, I will often ask him a question like, "Why are massage parlors such a trap for you?" This is typically when his head drops, as the old shame monster jumps on his back again. At this point, I will emphasize how infrequently he heard his dad openly affirm him and tell him how proud he was of him. Alternatively, he might have felt emotionally controlled by his mom. Now I am not saying his family of origin caused all of his destructive behavior. Mom and Dad probably did the best they could considering how they were raised. However, at some point, we need to stop the insanity of the generational curse. We need to take back what hell stole from us.

After asking the question, I will explain: "The reason massage parlors need to be in your inner circle and the reason you will always relapse when you go there is because you were starved of affirmation, and you have sexualized affirmation through human touch." Then I will lean forward and place my hand on his shoulder and declare to him, "Disengagement and isolation are the dirt in which lust always grows. God designed you to experience delight and tenderness from Mom and Dad. The problem is, in your home you were taught to live with a painful hunger in your heart; so you have sought to satisfy this need outside your home. You have continued to seek this in the home you are a part of now, but you will keep looking until you finally go off a cliff."

Your sexual acting out will be a direct reflection of your past which might include aspects of sexual abuse or neglect from your past. Here are some of the correlations I have noticed in over thirty years of counseling:

01. Men who have experienced a high level of abuse in their earlier years are far more likely to have an affair with someone they know.

02. Men who exhibit unaddressed anger, or as Dr. Carnes calls it, "erotized rage," experience a lot of sexual perversions such as voyeurism and exhibitionism.[120]

03. Men who seek out porn, which openly demeans women or is about having power over women, are often battling with very high levels of shame and frequently were raised by a strict father. It is interesting to note the vast majority of porn now falls into this category.[121]

04. Men who grew up in a home with little attention or affection from their mother can find themselves drawn to older women or fantasizing about older women and usually they have no understanding of why that vulnerability is present in their life.

The central factor I have found in all men's lives who are battling with pornography is an inability to see themselves from God's perspective; thus they have a profound lack of purpose in life. They have little, if any, experience with God's grace. They may have a theological or intellectual understanding of grace but have little or no understanding at the heart or limbic level. **Therefore, they can easily get trapped in the insanity of trying to get rid of pornography in their life by eliminating desire, instead of fighting to discover desire's meaning in their life. Sexual desire is a gift from God but hell has wounded us and distorted our desires so we will attempt to fulfill them in an illegitimate way.** Pornography is a symptom of a lack of God-given purpose in life and hell has injected a sense of futility in our soul.

As we wrap up this lesson, I want you to look back at your Arousal Template in Pillar 5 from *Seven Pillars of Freedom*. With the new information revealed in this chapter, look back at the work you did in Pillar 5 through the lens of grace and list the results of your observations below.

New Insights:

_____

_____

_____

_____

_____

_____

---

[120] Patrick Carnes, *Facing the Shadow: Starting Sexual and Relationship Recovery* (Carefree: Gentle Path Press, 2015), 333.

[121] Sam Carr, "How pornography removes empathy - and fosters harassment and abuse," *The Conversation*, November 1, 2017, https://theconversation.com/how-pornography-removes-empathy-and-fosters-harassment-and-abuse-86643.

What has driven your addiction?

If you struggle with relapses, in light of the new insights, what could you do to prevent relapses in the future?

In the last chapter, we discussed aspects of Jacob's life. However, most folks have little, if any, understanding of Esau's story and his amazing healing. He is usually dismissed as the idiot who sold his birthright for a bowl of soup!

Yet if you stop and read his story closely, you might see something most have never before noticed. Want to see it? **Esau made a life-changing decision that enabled him to walk in the blessings of God despite his family's betrayal.**

Look at Genesis 27:38-40 (NLT):

> *Esau pleaded, "But do you have only one blessing? Oh my father, bless me, too!" Then Esau broke down and wept.*
>
> *Finally, his father, Isaac, said to him, "You will live away from the richness of the earth, and away from the dew of the heaven above. You will live by your sword, and you will serve your brother. But when you decide to break free, you will shake his yoke from your neck."*

There is this fascinating moment when Esau is coming to meet Jacob with 400 warriors.[122] Jacob was convinced that Esau was going to pound him like a cheap steak and take everything he schemed so hard to obtain. When they met at the River Jabbok, however, Esau embraced him and declared he didn't need anything Jacob had because he was a blessed man.

---

[122] Genesis 32-33.

When you can embrace the person who betrayed you, then you no longer have a yoke around your neck!

For me, part of my healing happened when I was finally able to embrace my spiritual dad who betrayed me. The business administrator of the church we were part of stole over a million dollars. It turns out he was doing diamond deals with the mafia! It's the truth—you can't make this stuff up. I felt betrayed when the lead pastor, my spiritual dad, covered for the business administrator. This hurt me deeply, but by God's grace we were able to later repair the relationship.

We may have been betrayed by someone who is no longer around or someone who would not be safe to physically or emotionally embrace. But even in this situation, we can "embrace" them with grace before God and release their bondage from around our necks. We entrust the one who betrayed us to God, in order to move forward in our true identity.

I don't know if you have ever thought about this, but Esau must have wrestled with God long before Jacob ever did. We don't see it specifically delineated in Scripture, but there had to be a moment where Esau struggled with his identity. He may have been saying to himself, *I know what you have promised me, Lord. However, it doesn't look like it will ever happen because of what my father said to me and how my brother betrayed me!*

Somehow, he wrestled with God and wouldn't let go until he came to the understanding of who he was from God's perspective. He didn't receive validation from his dad or his brother or anyone else. He discovered he was who God said he was!

Like Valjean who came to believe the Bishop's words over him.

> *By the passion and the blood,*
> *God has raised you out of darkness:*
> *I have saved your soul for God!*[123]

Some of us here today need to come to the place of declaring to hell, "Even if no one ever knows my name, there is a God in heaven who knows me by name. I am more than enough in Him!"

Once you decide this is your truth, then the noose of not being enough and comparison will drop from your neck.

The only other option is to respond to the frustrations and wounds most of us experience in our dysfunctional families and say things like, "I didn't have a dad who ever told me I was good enough and I will never be like him."

---

[123] Colm Wilkinson, "The Bishop." Track 2 on *Les Misérables: The Motion Picture Soundtrack Deluxe*. Universal Music Group, 2013, CD.

I have heard this so many times in the counseling office. However, guess what you will grow up to be? A sucky dad just like he was! At some point in your life, you need to say:

> Lord, what do you have for me? I want to be obedient to You.
> Whatever You want to do through me—let it be!

Is it time for you to pray such a prayer? I double-dog dare you to open your heart and hands and express this prayer to God.

Write below what God has for you and what He wants to do through YOU!

_____
_____
_____
_____
_____
_____
_____
_____

Based on what you've learned so far, how is it helping you become a Compassionate Warrior? Be specific in your answer.

_____
_____
_____
_____
_____
_____
_____
_____

BE PREPARED TO SHARE WITH YOUR GROUP YOUR ANSWERS TO THE QUESTIONS IN THIS CHAPTER.

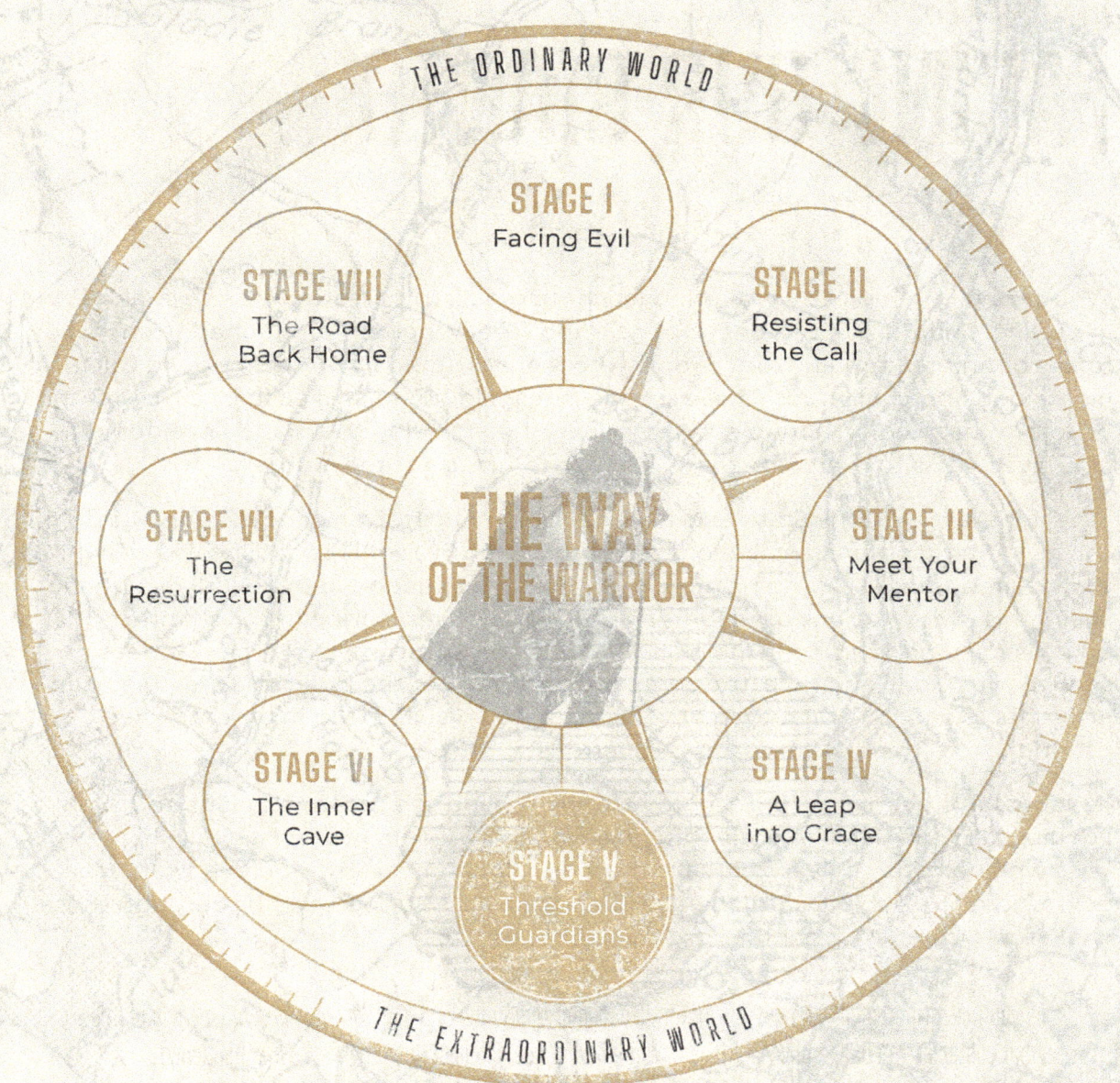

STAGE V

THRESHOLD GUARDIANS

CHAPTER 10
FACING OUR GIANTS

When we take a radical, life-altering leap into grace, this creates massive change in our life. Change like this does not go unnoticed. Whether intentionally from evil forces or unintentionally from people who feel disrupted by our change, we will face opposition and challenges. These are the threshold guardians; obstacles that tempt us to turn back before completing our quest. Recognizing them and developing effective tactics to overcome them is key to this stage of the journey.

Take, for example, Tony Stark in the Marvel Cinematic Universe movie, *Iron Man*.[124] In this film, Stark is a brilliant, billionaire playboy who lives only to satisfy his own whims and desires. After escaping from a deadly hostage situation in the Middle East—and seeing his own weapons used for terrorism—Stark feels compelled to change not only his personal mission in life, but his whole company as well. This move does not sit well with Obadiah Stane, the company president, or the Board of Directors. Stane attempts to destroy Stark, even developing his own suit of iron in order to keep profiting from the sale of weapons to terrorists.

It would have been easy for Stark to just turn a blind eye to Stane's plans and avoid conflict with him. Had he done this, however, Stark would never have become the hero who helped the Avengers save the world. In a similar way, you and I can back down from Threshold Guardians—it's the easier way! But persevering through these challenges is exactly what God uses to shape us!

> As you have experienced change in your life because of this group and your *Seven Pillars of Freedom* journey, what obstacles to change have you faced? Who or what has opposed this progress? What happened?

_____

_____

_____

_____

_____

[124] *Iron Man*, directed by Jon Favreau (Hollywood: Paramount Pictures, 2008), film.

In the Old Testament, Goliath's presence and comments triggered a massive fear response in the army of Israel. And his trash-talking put-downs of David immediately brought into question David's very worthiness to even be in the game. As David rushes toward Goliath, the Philistine mockingly cries out:

> *"Am I a dog, that you come at me with sticks?"*
> 1 SAMUEL 17:43 (NIV)

On the other hand, David's boldness in confronting Goliath demonstrates his sincere commitment to God's purposes in his life, which the conflict crystallizes for him. He was being tested at a deeply subconscious level. Fear is a limbic response triggered by our amygdala which is scanning the environment—between 12 to 100 times per second—for potential danger.[125] As the army of Israel hid in any foxhole they could find, they obviously picked up on the message the Philistine giant was broadcasting, loud and clear!

Combat can be a terrifying experience. I remember the first time I heard the North Vietnamese taunt us over the radio as we were flying in to provide air support for some besieged Marines. At the time, what made it particularly troubling was that I had no understanding of God's purposes in my life, so I eventually developed a tough guy exterior to try and ignore my inner fears.

For us to really begin to grasp God's purposes in our life we must grow in a healthy and dynamic balance in our times of revelation and meditation. Times of revelation are about us experiencing God. Times of meditation or hiddenness are different: they stem from the core of **our capacity to rest in the Lord**. We must develop the quietness of our heart and emotions before the Lord. Times of hiddenness in our life are when His presence is very much with us but we don't feel it in the same way.

God will love you enough to strip away all the external things in life that you continually look to for emotional support. In these challenging times, in the moment, you will need to *believe* you have peace with God—because you will not emotionally feel it. When we become comfortable with the ways of God in times of hiddenness, we will find ourselves going further in the realm of the Spirit than ever before. Why was David so bold in God? The power of his times of hiddenness are graphically described in 1 Samuel 17:

> *"Your servant has killed both the lion and the bear; this uncircumcised Philistine will be like one of them, because he has defied the armies of the living God. The Lord who rescued me from the paw of the lion and the paw of the bear will rescue me from the hand of this Philistine."*

---

[125] Méndez-Bértolo, C., Moratti, S., Toledano, R. et al. "A fast pathway for fear in human amygdala." *Nat Neurosci* 19, 1041–1049 (2016). https://doi.org/10.1038/nn.4324.

Saul said to David, "Go, and the Lord be with you."
1 SAMUEL 17:36-37 (NIV)

We would have never known about these events in David's life if Saul had not openly asked what makes him think he could take out this steroid overloaded Philistine. It was in the isolated years of caring for his family's flock that the groundwork was laid for David to come to an understanding of God's presence and purpose in his life. The purpose: he would be the next king of Israel.

Remember, David's dad hadn't even considered him as being remotely worthy of such an honor. After God told Samuel none of Jesse's sons who were lined up before him were to be king, the prophet turned to Jesse and asked him if he had any other sons. David's dad responded to the question in an amazing way, "There is still the youngest."[126] The NIV translated the Hebrew term qatan (pronounced "kaw-tawn") politely as youngest, but the term could also be translated as the "worthless one."

For David, on the day he confronted Goliath, all the times of hiddenness started to make sense. The pieces suddenly came together for him.

The same dynamic took place in the disciples' lives. After Jesus' Death, Burial, and Resurrection, suddenly things became crystal clear for the disciples. Much of what He had told them while they were enjoying His presence, they could not understand. But once He stood before them again in His resurrected state, things started to make sense.

"He will be delivered over to the Gentiles. They will mock him, insult him and spit on him; they will flog him and kill him. On the third day he will rise again." The disciples did not understand any of this. Its meaning was hidden from them, and they did not know what he was talking about.
LUKE 18:32-34 (NIV)

In hiddenness we discover our job is ultimately not to fight the devil. Our job is to "step back" into God and experience His majesty and power in the battles of life. Christ has overcome the devil so what we need to do is focus on being "in Christ."

You never need to go looking for the devil. If you live "in Christ," the devil will come and find you. In hiddenness God loves to tell you all about Himself but He wants to have **you all to Himself** to do this. If you are like me, these times of hiddenness can be the most challenging because it is so hard to "do nothing," like tending the flock. So often, I am running off to do something great for God; as a result, I miss the lesson of the lion and bear that God wants to teach me in private.

---

[126] 1 Samuel 16:11 (NIV).

How about you? How are you doing with your "hiddenness" in God? How are you taking regular time to rest in God and let Him strengthen you?

If you have taken times of hiddenness recently, what lessons have you gleaned?

If this is a struggle for you—or when it is—why is it? Why is taking time to rest in God hard for you?

It is also vital to understand that the Threshold Guardians we face in life are often God-given tests. And your gracious heavenly Father never gives you a test to fail but to equip you. In fact, it is impossible to fail any test God allows in your life. You know why? Because He will not just give it to you once—but again and again…and again…and again—until you pass it!

The toughest Threshold Guardians to deal with are not the external, chest-thumping Goliath types but the sinister, demeaning variety living within our own head.

I have few, if any, memories of my early childhood years because it was filled with so much abuse and violence. But there is one moment that resides at the very foundation of my sense of purpose in life; to this day, I can still remember it in vivid and brilliant colors. For some unknown reason, my mother and I were standing next to an airport and a fighter aircraft was taxiing by us prior to takeoff. I looked at my mom and unequivocally declared to her, "I am going to be a fighter pilot someday." I was only about 5 years old at the time.

It can be a real shock to your system to profoundly look at yourself from God's point of view. It can still bring tears to my eyes when I realize how God saw that five-year-old. This hit home for me through a series of events that happened much later as an adult. During the week prior to a Master Brainspotting Class[127] I had planned on attending, I experienced an extremely painful surgical procedure that involved very deep surgery on my nose. The surgeon had to cut so deeply on my nose to make sure he got all the cancer. The pain had reached the level where I didn't know if I could withstand any more! At that point, the doctors declared he would have to cauterize the area to stop the bleeding, which he was carving on! It was fine with me. I would try anything to deal with the pain.

What I didn't understand was this was a perfect situation for a Threshold Guardian to challenge me! The burning of human flesh has a very distinctive smell, and the moment he began cauterizing the wound, "BAM!" I was back in Vietnam; all the memories flooded my head again. Everything within me wanted to strike out and run but, somehow, I comprehended this was a spiritual battle that I could win by the grace of God. So I clenched my fists not to hit anyone but to stay steady and hold on to Christ.

Wait a minute, what does it have to do with seeing yourself as God sees you? Would you believe—EVERYTHING!

I had been profoundly disturbed by my flashback to Vietnam. This is why I shared my struggles with Dr. Grand during the Master Brainspotting Class the next week. You don't share your struggles with everyone but only with those who have earned the right to hear them. Dr. Grand is one of the wisest and most gracious men I have known. He listened to my story, then smiled and said, "Why don't you come up front and share with the class?" At that point, I was seriously questioning my assessment of him being so wise. I told him, "NO WAY!" There were 80 clinicians in the class. I was not going to share my struggles with all of them.

Somehow my trust in Dr. Grand was much greater than my fear of being rejected by 80 clinicians. As we started the session, Dr. Grand really caught me off guard with his first question, "Why did you become a fighter pilot?" I remember thinking, *What does this have to do with my nose*? But at the same time, the experience when I was five years old came flooding back to my memory. So I shared the declaration I had made to my mother that day so long ago, to which Dr. Grand responded with a very unique observation: "That was an amazing young man, wouldn't you say?"

I had never seen my five year old self as amazing in any way, but Dr. Grand's question caused me to pause and remember the innocence of my youth. And how deeply I

---

[127] Master Brainspotting Class. Brainspotting is an advanced brain-body technique for healing emotional trauma, anxiety, depression, and PTSD. It is one of the few techniques that effectively addresses the root cause of psychological stress and trauma. It is based on the premise that where you look, or your eye position, correlates with deep seated emotional experiences that are typically unreachable by traditional talk therapy.

loved God. There was also none of the cynicism that took root in my soul after my tour of duty in Vietnam. I just loved God and others and wanted everyone to encounter His amazing love.

The Brainspotting session continued for over an hour, as Dr. Grand walked beside me and helped me come to a new understanding of how deeply Christ loved that five-year-old boy. But Dr. Grand's next question truly floored me! No one had ever asked me such a question. He said, "What was the toughest part of dealing with your experiences in Vietnam?"

His loving but challenging questions caught me so off guard, I just responded to the question and didn't even try to make it sound acceptable. I found myself saying something that came from a dark place in my soul: "Killing the enemy wasn't something that I struggled much with. I guess I was just happy to be alive after a difficult mission." Then the tone of my voice changed and I remember my left hand trembling slightly as I said in a shaky voice, "The hardest part of serving in Nam was the experience of coming home and being spit upon in the San Francisco airport! I almost lost my mind for about two years."

Dr. Grand's face was filled with compassion as he leaned over and placed his hand on my shoulder. Then he said to me, "You are a hero." To which I vehemently responded, "I am no hero!" Dr. Grand wasn't changing his focus as he repeated his declaration, "You are a hero." And my response was even louder, "I AM NO HERO!" We both repeated our declarations two or three more times.

The tension in the room was suddenly broken, as 80 clinicians stood to their feet and gave me a standing ovation! This was the moment I totally lost it. I began to sob as I bent forward in my seat. This day, I faced my Threshold Guardian—my vicious inner critic—and finally saw myself the way God sees me.

God is repeatedly sending out casting calls for us to accept a starring role in our movie of the Hero's Journey for His glory. Then as we sit in the inner screening room of our life, we may wonder about the part we will need to play on this great stage of life. The surest way to discover your God-given destiny—in fact, the only way—is to begin to view yourself as God sees you!

Interestingly enough, in *The Matrix* movie, on a plaque over the Oracle's kitchen door, you may have noticed the statement in Latin, "Temet Nosce," meaning "Know Thyself."[128] In the film, Neo must first know himself before he can understand and be able to respond to the guidance he is receiving.

To live as a warrior for Christ we must ask ourselves the tough questions and challenge the status quo. Not examining ourselves might seem less painful but it is the coward's path to a slow and dull life. We can't avoid the ruthless questions the

---

[128] *The Matrix*, directed by Lana Wachowski and Lilly Wachowski (Burbank: Warner Bros, 1999), film.

Threshold Guardians will throw at us as we attempt to follow our dreams.

For me, the path to becoming a fighter pilot was not easy. I had just graduated from high school by the skin of my teeth and the dream of becoming a fighter pilot seemed totally impossible because there was no way I could get into college. My grade point average was abysmal, but they allowed me to take the entrance exams anyway. I totally failed the qualification exams and I had no financial support from my family. Beside all of this, I had the voices of several of my stepfathers roaring in my head saying things like, "You are a loser! You are stupid! Who told you, you could go to college?"

But I would not let go of the dream of becoming a fighter pilot despite the long odds I faced. I still remember living in my car for the first couple weeks of school and I could only afford one meal a day, so I ate at the local pancake house which advertised an "all you can eat special" for breakfast. Eventually, I was able to get several student loans and find work on campus. Of course, I had to take every "bonehead" class they offered so I could meet the academic entrance requirements. One day, I was sitting in the bonehead English class when I realized something about myself—I had a brain!

I went on to earn a 4.0 GPA that year and nearly every year after throughout my undergraduate schooling. The one exception was during the last part of my senior year in college. This was when I met my future wife. She was a huge distraction!

Without the Threshold Guardian of Goliath, David probably would not have recognized his call to be a warrior at such a young age. Without the Threshold Guardian of my inner critic, I would have never been forced to confront the demeaning voices in my head at such a critical stage in my life.

The Holy Spirit is always calling us to turn our **wounds** into **wisdom**.

It is in your true identity that the enemy of your soul seeks to deeply wound you. If you are wounded in the area of your God-given giftedness, your ability to invest in the things God has called you to in life is severely restricted. Your unresolved pain within will make you deeply self-focused. If you want to understand God's calling in your life, then you need to understand the places where you have been wounded in life. KNOW THYSELF!

> What dreams did you have as a young adult and what Threshold Guardians have you faced in life as a result of these dreams?

_____

_____

_____

_____

_____

What did you learn about yourself in the process of facing your Threshold Guardians?

How has facing your Threshold Guardians in other areas of your life prepared and equipped you to take on the Guardians you face now?

BE PREPARED TO SHARE WITH YOUR GROUP YOUR ANSWERS TO THE QUESTIONS IN THIS CHAPTER.

One of my good friends and coworkers, Robert Vander Meer, has done some beautiful work that relates to facing our Threshold Guardians. The next two chapters are his work, which will give you some powerful new insights into your story. He introduces a method he uses with clients, which he calls *The Superhero Odyssey*. This is only an overview of the approach, but I believe it will lead you to "know yourself" better than ever before!

CHAPTER 11
THE SUPERHERO ODYSSEY—PART 1

BY ROBERT VANDER MEER

"How can I be the hero if I need to ask for help?" This is what someone asked me several years ago during a counseling session. What a great question! Wrapped up in it were ideas about faith, value, trust, relationships, expectations, success, and failure.

That day as I continued to process the question, I realized all of us in some way or another face the same dilemma. Do we live as ourselves or try to be someone else? Do we face our pain and fear, or do we hide behind a facade? A mask? It feels safer to choose the mask. Better yet, some masks even come with capes. So we experience the safety that comes with hiding. We can escape our pain and fear while, at the same time, not feel weak. Thus, we develop our own superhero identity or personality. At first, most of us don't identify them as this. We just think we are funny, smart, a hard worker, giving, quiet, righteous, among other things, because this is how other people experience us. However, it's so much more than this.

From the conversation that day, I also noticed how these personalities all have similar narratives. For example, we experienced pain early in life. We developed ways to cope with this pain and our coping mechanisms became prominent in how we function. People attempt to get past the coping mechanisms or personality so they can get to know the real us, only to be turned away. We've all experienced "near death" moments where we realized we needed to change the way we were living or face desolate loneliness. We've had to make the choice of how we will live. The similarities were incredible to me. I started thinking about the superheroes I knew from graphic novels and movies. It seemed that most of them, if not all, also had similar stories—similar to each other and similar to ours.

Take for example, Bruce Wayne, aka Batman.[129] He saw his parents murdered in a back alley (early childhood pain). He was then raised by Alfred, a caretaker, and left

---

[129] DC Comics, "The Case of the Chemical Syndicate," *Detective Comics* #27, March 30, 1939, https://www.dc.com/blog/2019/03/19/batman-a-history-of-heroics-the-beginning.

only with the inherited wealth of his parents (pain continued). Afraid, he learned he could turn his own fear into a weapon and use it against others. Plus, he had lots of money to make cool gadgets (coping mechanisms). Women tried to get close to Bruce Wayne but he shut them out. Friends and mentors tried to get close to Bruce but, again, were not let in (people trying to get close). Over and over, he would run from his own fear and pain by turning it outward (more coping). Once being called the "Caped Crusader" but eventually known more appropriately as "The Dark Knight," we see an internal struggle between Bruce and Batman (more pain). Which one will he finally choose to live as? Villains come close to killing him (near death experiences). He wants to hang up his mask and cape to live as Bruce. He knows he will never have a family again if he continues as Batman (how will he live?). Gotham City needs Batman though. They need him to continue to protect it, and its people, from crime and villains. This is why Batman exists; because others need him. Or is it? Eventually we discover that Batman doesn't exist to protect Gotham. Ultimately, Batman exists to protect Bruce.

Just like *Iron Man* exists to protect Tony Stark.[130] Wolverine exists to protect Logan.[131] Even Clark Kent exists to protect Superman, his true identity.[132] In the end we are always left with the question, "Who will he decide to live as?" Will he decide to live as the protective identity, tormented and alone? Or will he decide to live as his true identity where relationships, family, and vulnerability are an option? To be continued…

The question goes unanswered. The internal conflict continues to be unresolved. This is why there have been 13 Batman movies since 1966; 14, if you include *The Lego Batman Movie* (which is my personal favorite).[133]

There's a scene in *The Lego Batman Movie* where Bruce is talking to Alfred, the family caretaker, where we get possibly the best insight into Bruce's internal conflict.[134]

> *Alfred: "Don't you think it's time you finally faced your greatest fear?"*
>
> *Bruce: "Snakes?"*
>
> *Alfred: "No."*
>
> *Bruce: "Clowns?"*

---

[130] Stan Lee, "Tales of Suspense #39," *Marvel Comics*, March 1963, https://ironman.fandom.com/wiki/Iron_Man%27s_Comics.

[131] John Romita, "The Incredible Hulk #180," *Marvel Comics*, October 1974, https://tvtropes.org/pmwiki/pmwiki.php/ComicBook/Wolverine.

[132] Jerry Siegel, "The Reign of the Superman," January 1933, https://www.history.com/news/8-things-you-may-not-know-about-superman.

[133] *The Lego Batman Movie*, directed by Chris McKay (Burbank: DC Entertainment, 2017), film.

[134] *The Lego Batman Movie*.

Alfred: "No."

Bruce: "Snake-clowns?"

Alfred: "Bruce, listen. Your greatest fear is being a part of a family again." (Long pause where Bruce looks at a family photo. It appears he is going to admit what he really is afraid of...)

Bruce: "Nope. Now it's snake-clowns because you put that idea in my head. Time for push-ups! One...two...were going to 1,000. I'm already at 20."

The reality of our common narratives led me to create "*The Superhero Odyssey.*" In the next two chapters we are going to look at how each of us, as a result of our experiences, develop and nurture "superhero" personalities. We will walk through identifying and naming your own personal superhero while also identifying the Threshold Guardians that you encounter along the way.

Who or what is a Threshold Guardian? The Threshold Guardian, one of the characters from The Way of the Warrior, stands at the gateway to a new world or adventure. Their job is to test the hero and make sure they are worthy and ready to advance to the next stage. In literature and movies, they do this in a variety of ways. In some cases, they work for the villain and the hero must fight their way past to prove their strength. In other cases, they are a neutral figure who simply presents a riddle or challenge. Sometimes, they are a friend who has come to rely on some aspect of the hero and, thus, doesn't want them to move on to the next stage. In all scenarios they are testing the hero's desire and ability to move on.

In this chapter and the next, we will identify the threshold as being the moment when the hero/superhero is faced with the question: "Who will you be? Your superhero identity or your true identity?" In our process of recovery, it is the question of "**Will you continue to live in fear and cope the way you have learned? Or will you face your fear and attempt to trust again?**"

We will identify several moments in your narrative where you approached the threshold only to be defeated by the Guardian. With each defeat you became more dependent on your superhero identity and yet more desperate to change. Until finally...

...to be continued.

The Birth of a Superhero

My wife, Rebecca, and I used to live in San Isidro; a small town just outside of Buenos Aires, Argentina, where every year there was a festival that celebrated cinema and music. The way the festival worked was every night for a week, a different movie was played outdoors at a different location. The cool part, though, was that all of the movies were black-and-white silent films and were accompanied by live music performed during the screening. The first movie we went to see was the 1939 version of *The Hunchback of Notre Dame*.[135] We sat in chairs that were set up on the cobblestone street just outside of a Catholic Cathedral. It was definitely one of the most memorable movie experiences I've ever had. The lighting, camera angles, facial expressions, and music all came alive together to create and deliver a message that didn't require the sound of a human voice.

Every night that week we went to see a different movie and were equally captivated by each unfolding storyline. No spoken words were needed to understand how each character moved through their own story and eventually arrived at the end. The lighting at the beginning of the scene would start our minds going with anticipation. The camera angle would make us lean in our chair to try and see around the corner of the hallway where we thought the villain might be lurking. The music would make our hearts race with excitement, not knowing what would happen next. So much storytelling was possible with what seemed like so little. It was amazing what lighting, camera angles, and music could do to add to a story and help us feel what the characters were experiencing.

In the same way, the dim lighting of the Batcave lets us know that Batman isn't just a mysterious part of Bruce Wayne but also a sad and dark one. Or the bright lighting of Tony Stark's lab isn't just about making robotics but it's also a way for Tony to feel like his life isn't always on the precipice of losing everything. You could say we are reading into these things, but this is exactly the way cinema works.

In this chapter, we're going to begin working through scenes of your life. But we don't just want the description of the events, we want the Hollywood version with lighting, camera angles, dialogue, and even a soundtrack. In doing this you can add to your own stories a feeling that, quite possibly, you've never been able to articulate. Once your scene is written, you can sit back and observe your own story unfold before you; almost as if you were sitting in the balcony of a theater watching a play. This puts you into a position called the "objective observer." By watching your own story in this objective way, it gives you the ability to understand the plight of the main character, you, and even maybe have empathy and grace where there was once only judgment and shame. It will also help you to see more clearly the role and impact of Threshold Guardians, which we will unpack mainly in Part 2.

SCENE 1:

In this scene, you will need to think back to a painful **early childhood** memory. The earlier the better in terms of setting the stage for the rest of the story. Write down what happened: who was involved; how it made you feel.

---

[135] *The Hunchback of Notre Dame*, directed by William Dieterle (Culver City: RKO Radio Pictures, 1939), film.

NOTE: As you are going through this chapter you will be asked to think about pain from your past and it may hurt. Our goal isn't to make you hurt for the sake of pain. Our goal is that you will be able to have a coherent narrative and move toward a greater understanding of yourself, your past, your present, and your possible future. Please reach out to someone during this exercise so you are not processing through these memories alone.

Next, take this same memory and begin "Hollywoodizing" it. What time of day did the scene start? What was the lighting like? What camera angle would you use to start the scene? Are there sounds in the background, like birds chirping or children playing? What are the other people in the scene doing? Is there dialogue? Is there a soundtrack? After the painful experience, what does the main character do? How does the scene end? Does the camera pan out or fade to black? Don't be afraid to embellish. Embellishments help to communicate the feelings involved in the scene and with the characters involved.

Here's an example of Scene 1 from someone else's story.

PAINFUL CHILDHOOD MEMORY:

Sunny outside, although the scene is set in the living room. House is a fairly plain, single-story brick house. The driveway is on the right. The grass outside is mostly brown due to intense heat and lack of rain. The living room has cream colored carpet, a brown coffee table, a blue couch, and a huge TV in an entertainment center.

Start Underoath's song *To Whom It May Concern*.[136] The first scene opens to the song at 0:00. The scene begins with an aerial view of the house for a few seconds, birds are heard chirping and a light wind is noticed. The camera then fades to a view from the kitchen, looking into the living room. His dad is zoned out looking at the TV. A young boy, maybe seven years old, is drinking milk from a boot-shaped glass mug. He places the glass on the table. The camera zooms in very close and as the glass makes contact with the table, the song reaches 2:29.

For the next 25 seconds, you see the boy playing with his toys. Suddenly, as the young boy is playing, he accidentally knocks over the glass of milk, causing it to spill all over the table and onto the carpet. At that exact moment, the whole scene becomes slow motion as the song hits 2:50, 2:51, 2:52, 2:53. The camera focuses on the child's face which shows a horrific fear. He knows he just woke the giant. At 2:54 of the song, the dad stands up and yells, "Why do you act like a jackass!" The child stands up and begins running out of fear, the dad closes on his tail like a lion to a gazelle. The boy runs circles around the coffee table,

---

[136] Spencer Chamberlain, "*To Whom It May Concern*." Track 11 of *Define the Great Line*. Tooth & Nail Records, 2006, CD.

only to be snatched by his arm. At this moment, the camera transitions to blurry; the song is around 4:30. You see movement but you're not sure whether the dad is just yelling or also spanking the child. You hear the lyrics on the song "At the end of the road, you'll find what you've been longing for."[137]

The camera fades to black.

Take some to capture the details that come to mind from your story including the setting, the lighting, camera angles, and sounds. What song is playing in your story?

Time to write your own Scene 1. Use extra paper if you would like.

---

[137] Spencer Chamberlain, "*To Whom It May Concern*."

SCENE 2:

Now that you're getting warmed up, let's move on to scene 2. Think back to a painful memory from your **teenage years**. Work through the scene with the same steps you did with Scene 1.

Here's an example of Scene 2 from someone else's story.

PAINFUL TEENAGE MEMORY:

Scene is from Donald's point of view (through his eyes): dark, opening eyes; dark, opening eyes; dark, opening eyes but distorted, like looking through water (tears). The next camera angle is showing him in his bedroom sitting on his bed. He has a distant stare as he wipes tears from his eyes. He painfully remembers a memory that he tries to push aside every day, but it keeps returning.

The scene becomes blurry and transitions to Donald in the dormitory at football camp. He hates football camp. Not only is it horrendous physical strain from 5:00 am to 10:00 pm every day for a week, but the worst is having to deal with Mickey, Joe, Brad, Jay, Joel, Jeremy, and all the other guys who make fun of him every day. One day in between camp practices, Mickey is taunting Donald more aggressively than normal. He's mocking him while all the others are laughing. Donald keeps his head down trying to dodge each comment. Mickey asks, "Hey, I bet you would kiss Smith's butt for $10!" Everyone is laughing and pointing at Donald, making motions with their mouths. Donald snaps back "Shut up, Mickey!" Mickey then states, "Fine. How about $25?" Donald yells, "SHUT UP, Mickey!" Finally, he says "Okay, okay, okay. But surely you'd kiss his butt for $50, right?" Donald can't stand it, puts his head down, and walks out of the room. As he walks out, Mickey yells, "$50 it is! He would kiss his butt for $50!"

The Champion and His Burning Flame plays a song, *Redemptron x 7*.[138] The song begins at 0:00 and fades out at 0:55.

---

[138] The Champion and His Burning Flame, "Redemptron x 7." Track 2 on *Song & Film*. Distant Second Music, 2009, CD.

Time to write your own Scene 2. Notice in the above two scenes, at the most painful moment, the camera focus goes blurry. This is a great way to identify a common thread in the main character's experience. Try to find something similar in your story. Could be going blurry, the sound becoming muted, a light flickering, or a dog barking. This will help you to see how these experiences are not totally separate. The main character, you, is facing a defining pain in multiple scenarios that will wound him for a long time to come.

SCENE 3:

At this point in the main character's life, pain has become woven into the storyline. Though you have only written two scenes, if this was a movie you were watching, you would already have a picture of the challenges that lie ahead for the main character. Pain is unavoidable.

A quick side note: don't compare your story with anyone else's story. Your pain is your pain. If you remember the moments from the first two scenes, it's because they left an impact. It's easy for us to minimize our experiences and brush them aside as no big deal. But again, if your same painful moments were in a movie or book, you wouldn't think twice about the obvious impact they had.

So, what did you start doing to no longer feel the pain? Did you become a funny guy, try to be attractive, smart, or a hard worker? Did you take all of that pain and stuff it down until you exploded with anger on those around you? Did you procrastinate until the last moment and then dazzle everyone with what you were able to accomplish in so little time? Did you hide in sports or the outdoors? Did you turn toward a perfectionist approach to religion? Did life become about value through performance?

Use the space below to make a list of the things you did to avoid pain in your life. Then choose the one you did the most or was the most powerful. Whatever it was, this became your superpower. For this exercise, choose something other than your sexual addiction. The reality is, you probably have some other coping mechanism you use even more frequently than your sexual behavior. Possibly, like one of the things I mentioned.

How I avoid pain in life: (Make a list; then, circle the most frequent or powerful behavior.)

▸ _____
▸ _____
▸ _____
▸ _____
▸ _____
▸ _____
▸ _____
▸ _____
▸ _____

My Superhero Identity: _____

Think back to a time when you remember using this strategy (superpower) to deal with pain. Use this experience to write Scene 3. Hollywoodize it and come up with a superhero identity.

Here's an example of Scene 3 from someone else's story.

WAYS TO AVOID PAIN AND THE BIRTH OF A SUPERHERO:

List of things he did to avoid pain:

- Feats of strength
- Commanding physical presence
- Words have "magical" powers
- Speaks to the desires of women

He realized he did all of these things as a way to try and impress people and find value. He named his superhero identity "Mr. Charisma."

Mr. Charisma doesn't truly earn his name until he grows from his early teenage years to his later teenage years. Even when attacked by the Evil Ones (the guys who picked on him in Scene 2), with their best efforts to turn even random bystanders against him, Mr. Charisma is still able to smile the right way, flirt the right way with girls, and make humorous comments to hopefully gain positive attention from anyone he could. His acne clears as he gains more maturity. Suddenly, Mr. Charisma is considered one of the most attractive guys at school. When all is said and done, Mr. Charisma tries his hardest to make people laugh and convince them he has it all together and doesn't cry every night alone in his bed.

Another one of his superpowers is his ability to release energy on the football field: a stronger energy than anyone else. This energy is partly through internal power and partly from anger (though he's not willing to admit it). The camera angle shows Mr. Charisma on the football field. He's the starting defensive end and recently learned the other team studies his every move, trying their best to figure out how to beat him but they never do. The ball snaps and he just crushed the running back. See, Mr. Charisma has always been able to impress people on the field; both bystanders and sometimes even the Evil Ones. When everything was a struggle in his life, when things were falling apart, he could release one of these secret powers of being faster, more agile, and a harder hitter than everyone else on the team. The camera zooms in on the ball. The moment the ball snaps, Mr. Charisma cuts through the offensive line and sacks the quarterback. He immediately hops up, initially looking at the quarterback who's in agonizing pain, but then looking to the crowd to hear the fan's scream his name. The cheering by the crowd is partially fulfilling but you see his eyes scanning the crowd to see his father...he's not there.

Time to write your own Scene 3. Remember to embellish the truth here. Take real events where you avoided pain with whichever strategy applies to you and add the Hollywoodized version where your superpower kicks in. Keep using camera angles, lighting, music, and more to capture the feeling of the scene.

Congratulations, you're a superhero! Bummer though, you've also effectively discovered one of the multiple ways you will diligently work to avoid pain over the next years of your life.

It's easy to tell ourselves that the superhero is there to help others. This is how it often appears on the outside. The reality is, however, that the superhero exists not to protect Gotham, **but to protect himself**. The entire creation and perpetuation of this new identity is centered on keeping you from feeling pain. The pain of loss, family, failure, loneliness, embarrassment, and most of all shame. Shame tells us that no matter how hard we try, there is no safe place for us to just simply be ourselves. So, to ensure the need and existence of the alter ego, where we don't have to face our shame, we begin to be hypervigilant. We are constantly on the lookout for an excuse to put on our cape and mask and hide in safety.

Here is an interesting thought. Who was it that was always on the lookout for the Batsignal? Batman or Bruce Wayne? It was Bruce Wayne. He was always hypervigilant, keeping one eye toward the night sky because it felt safer for him to hide from his own pain and fear as Batman than it did for him to face his loneliness as Bruce Wayne.

> " Being alone is scary, but not as scary as feeling alone..."[139]

In the next chapter, we will introduce the Threshold Guardian into your Superhero Odyssey. It's probably not the Guardian you were expecting, but it's definitely the most difficult one to get past. In the meantime, check-in with someone and process through the things you just discovered about yourself and your own storyline.

But by the grace of God I am what I am, and his grace toward me was not in vain.
1 CORINTHIANS 15:10 (ESV)

BE PREPARED TO SHARE WITH YOUR GROUP YOUR ANSWERS TO THE QUESTIONS IN THIS CHAPTER.

---

[139] Amelia Earhart, Gracious Quotes, *52 Inspiring Amelia Earhart Quotes*, September 14, 2022, https://graciousquotes.com/amelia-earhart/.

CHAPTER 12
THE SUPERHERO ODYSSEY—PART 2

BY ROBERT VANDER MEER

The Death of a Superhero and the True Threshold Guardian

At this point, you've laid the groundwork for your backstory, as well as identified your superhero identity. Through your painful moments, you've begun to see a common thread connecting your experiences and pain. Organically, you've seen how there is a theme rising out of your story—one of pain, fear, failure, loss, and, most painful of all, loneliness. Out of this pain, you have learned how to survive using the tools at hand, working with what you have been given. Most of these tools are effective in the short term for keeping away the truth of your unwanted reality but in the long term leading to isolation. In the mix of these tools, you found something that works for you above all else. It is your go-to. It is the thing you have come to depend on more than friendship and God. It is your superhero identity.

With this identity, you have discovered you can avoid pain, fear, failure, and loneliness. You have found a way to hide in plain sight and eventually be celebrated by those around you. You've fooled them and even begun to fool yourself with the delusions that this superhero identity is needed and possibly even really who you were created to be. You've come to believe this is who you are. So now what?

Now enters the Threshold Guardian. If you remember, the Threshold Guardian is the one who stands at the gateway to growth, advancement, change, development, adventure, and intimate relationships. It stands there to test you to see if you are really ready for the next stage of the journey. If you fail the test, then you don't advance. You stay stuck, stagnant, and arrested in your development. The greatest of all Threshold Guardians is one who we have come to identify in the recovery process. It doesn't speak to our failures, but it calls to the deepest parts of how we see ourselves and says, "You ARE a failure." It is known by the name, "Shame." This shame can come to us from external sources or from our own internal dialogue. Usually, it's a combination of both.

As you develop the next several scenes of your Superhero Odyssey you will see how the Threshold Guardian, Shame, is there to meet you and test how serious you are about moving on with your life and relationships. Will you choose the risk and fear that comes with being yourself or will you stay behind the safety of a false personality? I should note, **taking the risk of being yourself is one of the greatest risks you can take**. Because what if you are yourself and no one likes you? What if you are honest with your feelings, thoughts, desire, and failures, and you are rejected for these things? Taking the risk to embrace yourself and allow others to see you is a scary thing. But if you don't face this risk, you can't find peace, fulfillment, relationship, or joy. You can only find the fabricated reality you've been living in.

Living as yourself requires facing fear. If you aren't willing to interact with fear, you can't interact with people or God. Having a healthy relationship with God and people necessitates a healthy relationship with fear. This includes the fear of facing our shame.

SCENE 4:

In this scene, you will need to think back to a time when you had a close relationship with a friend or mentor. In this relationship, you had the opportunity to become even closer and let them get to know the real you, but instead you backed away. Maybe you began to let them know your true identity only to realize it wasn't safe. Or maybe they tried to get close but you immediately shut them out by keeping it surface level and only talking about sports, church, work, or motorcycles. In this experience, you were close to living as yourself, but Shame showed up and told you it wasn't worth it because they wouldn't like who you are.

Here's an example of Scene 4 from someone else's story.

A FRIEND TRIES TO GET CLOSE TO THE REAL YOU. YOU DON'T LET THEM IN.

In his later high school years, Donald/Mr. Charisma befriends a man named Jon. Jon and Mr. Charisma play in a band together, covering worship songs, Dave Matthews, Jack Johnson, and Switchfoot songs. See, Jon and Mr. Charisma spend hours and hours together. They would fish, smoke, party, and drive for hours in Mr. Charisma's jeep. Jon seems different though. He's always the one to recommend playing a worship song. Mr. Charisma seems distant from this draw to God. While on vacation, Jon asks Mr. Charisma to go sit on a dock over the Beaufort River and play worship songs. As much as Mr. Charisma has become dear friends with Jon, he can't be broken through. He doesn't want to open up and become vulnerable to a "God" who has let him down so many times in the past; but believes deep within that he was actually the one letting God down.

Jon leaves and walks down to the dock to spend time with God. Mr. Charisma walks to the campsite, lights a cigarette, and falls asleep within a short time.

Mr. Charisma never knew this but Jon looked up to him. Years later, as Mr. Charisma draws closer to God, Jon abandons Him. Mr. Charisma seems to have missed out on an opportunity. Donald almost let in Jon and God. But in the end, he didn't believe that who he was would be accepted and wasn't willing to be hurt again. The Threshold Guardian told him it wasn't worth it and instead of wrestling with Shame, he lowered his head and returned to live as Mr. Charisma.

Donald didn't make it past the Threshold Guardian of Shame and, at some point in your story, neither did you.

Time to write your own Scene 4.

SCENE 5:

This fifth scene is similar to the last. However, instead of a friendship or mentor you kept at arm's length, this time think about a romantic relationship. It could be a relationship that never even got started because you were unwilling and unable to take a risk. Or maybe you got the relationship started, went on dates, looked longingly at each other, but then you realized in these feelings you also might get hurt. So, you shut it down and put up a wall. She might have still married you but you haven't ever really let her in. Write about it here. The time you almost took off your mask and cape for a girl. Again, you had a chance for something new and exciting. You could have loved and been loved. Towering at the threshold of love was Shame. It stood tall and told you, "You can't open up to her. You'll never be enough. She'll reject you if she really knew you."

Here's an example of Scene 5 from someone else's story.

A WOMAN TRIES TO GET CLOSE TO THE REAL YOU. YOU DON'T LET HER IN.

> It's now a couple years after fighting the Evil Ones. He left their village to try to regain his identity. He meets the most amazing and beautiful woman in the world and has no idea it will be the biggest challenge he'll ever face. Her name is Laura. She has red hair, down to the middle of her back. It's curly and waves behind her like a blanket of red gold. Her smile is glowing and her voice attracts Mr. Charisma like a Siren to Odysseus. Yet Laura causes no harm. She builds him up the best she can. He wins her and they marry.
>
> Mr. Charisma opens himself up to Laura as much as he can but doesn't realize how his past battles have crippled him to deep relationships. Laura trusts Mr. Charisma. She gives him her heart, her mind, her soul but he has no idea how to protect these things. Over the years, he keeps her at arms length. She tries and tries to get close but he pushes her away. Instead of connecting physically with her, he turns to artificial beauty. Despite having the most real relationship so close to him, he chooses fake, worthless, and unfulfilling connections. He wonders what the future holds and whether this marriage is what it's supposed to be.

Donald was close but he didn't make it past Shame's powerful voice. He couldn't; he was too scared. Fear held him back and it held you back too.

Time to write your own Scene 5.

SCENE 6:

All superheroes face a near-death experience. It's the moment when their powers weren't as strong as they thought they were. The time when the opponent's strength was too much and regardless of how hard the superhero fought, he kept... getting... knocked... down...

Think of your own "near-death" experience. For most people, this was the lowest moment of their life. When all of their attempts at success failed. When their talent and skill could no longer span the gap between who they really were and who they pretended to be. They lost friendships, jobs, ministries, marriages, possessions. This was their rock bottom. Emotionally they were wrecked. What was this moment for you? How did your superpower let you down?

In this moment, you stood (more like laid curled up in the fetal position) at the threshold of change. You were broken. But was the pain enough for you to fight past the Guardian of Shame to do one last heroic act? Was the desperation enough to lead you to muster up the courage and strength to heroically ask for help?

Here's an example of Scene 6 from someone else's story.

NEAR-DEATH EXPERIENCE:

It's been five years since Mr. Charisma married Laura. They maintain a decent relationship, although shaky at times due to Mr. Charisma's anger problem. He can't describe or explain why he feels anger. He wonders if it has to do with his father or the Evil Ones, but quickly throws the thought in the trash. It seems too painful to think about.

Mr. Charisma, although having Laura, continues to seek an artificial connection. Although now an addiction, his desire to connect with the artificial has moved from two dimensional to three: he meets The Heroin. She has a superpower that she doesn't realize draws Mr. Charisma to her. This fake connection is everything Mr. Charisma wants and feels will fulfill him. At this point in his life, his superpower is stronger than ever. It no longer takes weeks and months to turn a woman on to him. It is now only a few text messages. She makes it clear that she finds him handsome, funny, and overall sexy. Mr. Charisma realizes he's never even been called sexy. The Heroin, only called that by Mr. Charisma, gained her name by being one of the most addictive things he has ever faced. He tries his hardest to resist but continues to return to her.

While driving together one day, he lets her use one of her special powers on him. As the experience happens, Mr. Charisma convinces himself this is what he deserves and this will definitely make him feel more like a man. He never knew that The Heroin didn't truly want him. She was only medicating her own hurt, fears, and traumas. He thought his powers had drawn her in; but in reality, his powers had failed him and he was the one being played.

Laura discovers the relationship. Mr. Charisma tries his hardest to keep her and through his false, empty words he convinces her to stay. But he doesn't realize that without addressing his deepest secrets and traumas, these horrific moments will only continue to happen.

His pain is excruciating. The Threshold Guardian, Shame, stands before him again telling him that he is a failure and a disappointment. He not only feels alone but feels he is alone in the world. No one wants him or will love him if they really find out. He should run. He should hide. He should keep trying to use his powers to lure more women; defeat more opponents; impress his coworkers and pastors.

Some superheroes experience multiple near-death experiences. Will your experience be the starting point of choosing your true identity; or will the bottom drop out further and he, you, will be forced to experience more pain before asking for help?

Time to write your own Scene 6. What has been your superhero's near-death experience?

SCENE 7 A & B:

I hope you asked for help. We're going to find out in this final scene with alternate endings. These final scenes will be based not on something that has happened, but on something that will happen. Think into the future and write two separate endings to this story. What does life look like **15 years** from now? In the first ending, write what life looks like 15 years from now if you choose to continue to hide behind your superhero mask and avoid the Threshold Guardian. Shame has defeated you and you continue to run toward isolation and addiction. You have no close friends. Your marriage, if you have one, is a farce. You still have not made it past the Threshold Guardian.

Start this scene with the words, "Because of my superhero identity…"

Here's an example of Scene 7a from someone else's story.

LIVING AS YOUR SUPERHERO IDENTITY 15 YEARS FROM NOW:

Because of my superhero identity…Mr. Charisma is now in his 40s. Laura finally had enough. She was hurt too many times. He refused to ever let her into his heart. He always pushed her away and would use his superpower to seek other pleasures. He doesn't realize it but his superpower has now weakened. He doesn't seem to have as much strength as in the past. He wonders if he will eventually die…until he does die. He abandoned all friends, family, real relationships and, most importantly, God. He chose his superpower over the real power of God. His grave is unmarked and the only one to know its location is his mother and Laura, but neither visit often. At one point, his mother and Laura visit together…tears falling down their faces. All you hear is them screaming, "Why Donald? Why couldn't you let down your guard? Why couldn't you have given yourself to God, to family, to real relationships?" They leave and the camera fades to black.

9 Crimes by Damien Rice plays in the background:[140]

> *Leave me out with the waste*
> *This is not what I do*
> *It's the wrong kind of place*
> *To be thinking of you*
> *It's the wrong time*
> *For somebody new*
> *It's a small crime*
> *And I've got no excuse…*
> *It's the wrong kind of place*
> *To be cheating on you…*

---

[140] Damien Rice, "9 Crimes." Track 1 on 9. 14th Floor Records, 2006, CD.

Time to write your own first ending of Scene 7.

Because of my superhero identity…

_____
_____
_____
_____
_____
_____
_____
_____
_____
_____
_____
_____

In the second ending, write what life looks like if you choose to live as yourself. Did you finally get close to that friend or mentor? Did you allow yourself to love and be loved? Were you willing to face fear and, therefore, open up to the possibility of receiving and experiencing God's love and grace? If you defeated Shame as a Threshold Guardian, then the answer to these questions is "yes." You have moved on and are striving to live as your God-created identity.

Start this ending with the phrase, "Because of the kind of person I am…"

Here's an example of Scene 7b from someone else's story.

LIVING AS YOUR TRUE IDENTITY 15 YEARS FROM NOW:

Because of the kind of person I am…Mr. Charisma, now known as Donald, lives a different life. He is in his late 60s. You see Donald and Laura sitting in chairs in the backyard of their home. Their daughter, Beautiful, and her husband sit on the patio with them as Donald's grandchildren play in the backyard. You see smiles on everyone's face. Donald now knows how to connect with reality. He has no need for the fake world: the world that doesn't fulfill; the world that leaves one empty. He is happier than ever, full of love from The Father. He speaks with his mom and dad daily and has a strong relationship with them.

The last scene is Donald looking toward his children and you see Laura looking at Donald. She is living in heaven on earth. Her hero is home. He bows to The Father every morning before then pouring into her and the children. Donald is brighter now. The darkness is gone. The heaviness is gone.

She smiles with tears of peace falling down her cheeks.

In the background, David Crowder sings an acoustic version of *O Praise Him*:[141]

> *Oh, the sound of salvation come*
> *The sound of rescued ones*
> *And all this for a king*
> *Angels join to sing*
> *All for Christ our King!*
>
> *O praise Him!*
> *O praise Him!*
> *He is Holy!*
> *He is Holy!*

Time to write your own second ending of Scene 7.

Because of the kind of person I am...

---

[141] David Crowder Band, "O Praise Him (All This for a King)." Track 3 on *Illuminate*. SixstepsRecords, 2003, CD.

You've been on an odyssey your whole life. You can't look at today removed from the context of this odyssey. Piecing together all of these scenes it's easy to see how you ended up where you are today. It makes sense. You experienced pain, everyone does. (If you skipped these chapters because you can't identify pain, keep working and looking. If you have no pain, you have no need for Jesus. This is a scary thought.)

During your odyssey you discovered ways to avoid your pain, thus adopting a sort of superhero identity. Again and again you tried to break free from its confines and move on to the next stage but you were unable because of the most powerful of all Threshold Guardians: Shame. Hopefully you've begun the process of moving beyond this threshold.

The reality is, we never really defeat shame until we die. Jesus defeated its eternal effect in His Death and Resurrection. This is called justification. However, we have to continue to fight it, threshold after threshold, for the rest of our lives. This is called sanctification. Having been justified, we are all being sanctified; which means God isn't expecting perfection from you. Perfection is in Jesus. He is expecting progress, however. Progress and not perfection.

Keep fighting Shame when it shows its ugly head. You'll get better at it with practice. It won't hold you back the way it used to. Have grace for your superhero when he shows up to try and help. He was there for a long time to try and help you to survive. In fact, he did help you to survive. You need to live as yourself now. There is only one of you and the most important thing you can bring into a room is yourself, in your God-given identity. Christ in you.

When Paul was questioned for his less than stellar past he said,

> *But whatever I am now, it is all because God poured out his special favor on me—and not without results. For I have worked harder than any of the other apostles; yet it was not I but God who was working through me by his grace.*
> 1 CORINTHIANS 15:10 (NLT)

Progress and not perfection.

How has this exercise helped you understand the Threshold Guardian you currently face?

_____
_____
_____
_____
_____
_____

How does your storyline up to this point inform the decision(s) you need to make next in order to keep moving forward on The Way of the Warrior?

In addition to Shame, you may still be facing additional Threshold Guardians. Write out scenes (7A and B) for other present examples of these Guardians in your life. *Examples: Secrecy, Isolation, Self-Absorption, Managing your reputation, Finding your identity through performance or success.*

Based on what you've learned so far, how is it helping you become a Compassionate Warrior? Be specific in your answer.

BE PREPARED TO SHARE WITH YOUR GROUP YOUR ANSWERS TO THE QUESTIONS IN THIS CHAPTER.

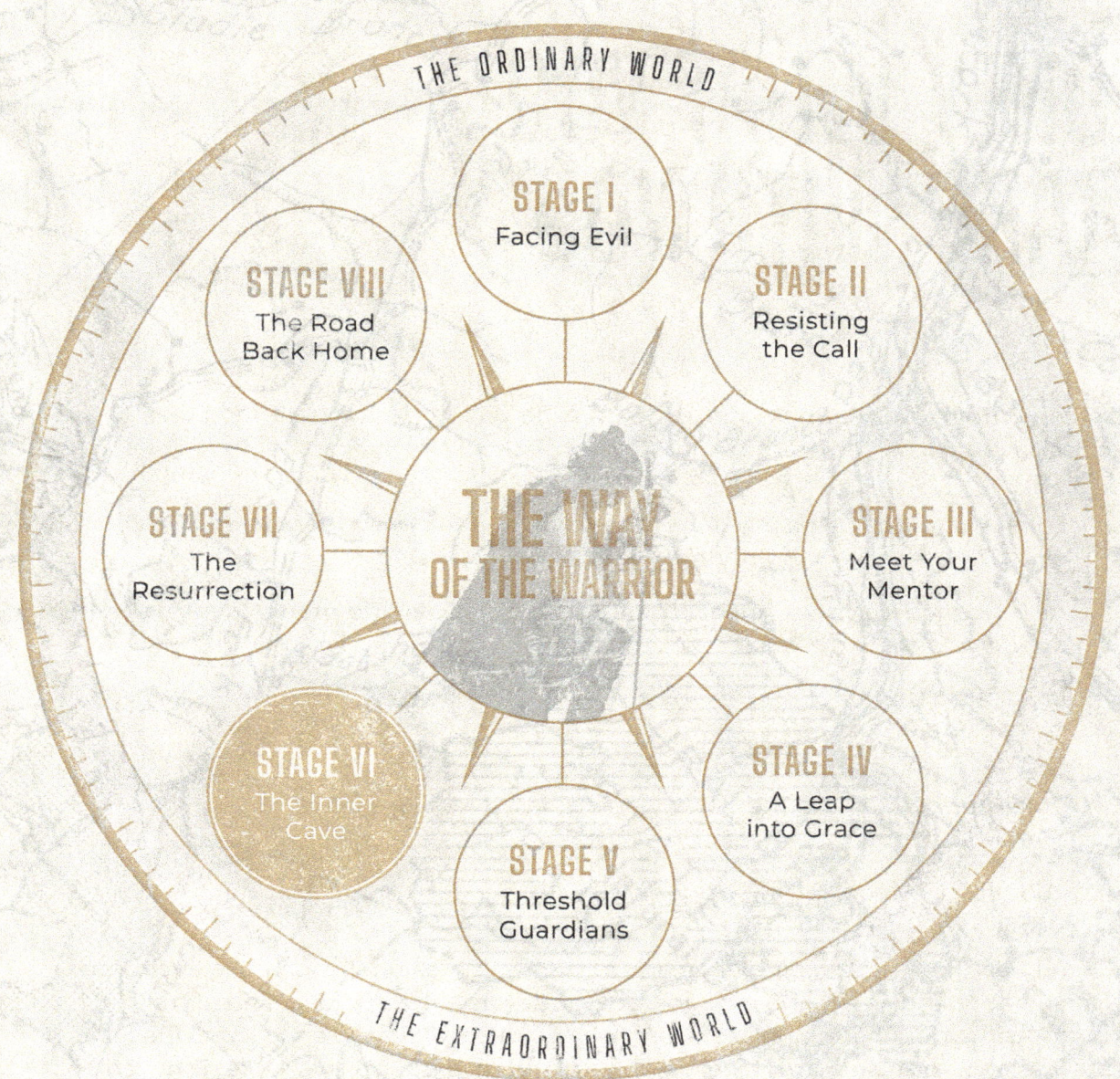

STAGE VI
THE INNER CAVE

CHAPTER 13
ONLY WHAT YOU TAKE WITH YOU

In *The Empire Strikes Back: Star Wars* Episode V, as Yoda is mentoring Luke, we find a classical picture of facing the Inner Cave:[142]

> *Luke was suddenly distracted. He sensed something dangerous, something evil. "There's something not right here…I feel cold. Death."*
>
> *As he turned he saw a huge, tangled tree…the roots had grown to form the opening to a darkly sinister cave.*
>
> *Luke felt a tremor of apprehension. "What's in there?"*
>
> *"Only what you take with you," Yoda said cryptically.*
>
> *Luke stepped toward the dark opening between those great and foreboding roots.*
>
> *Yoda responded, "Your weapons…you will not need them."*

Yet, Luke ignores Yoda's guidance and takes his lightsaber. Inside Luke encounters Darth Vader and, in a terrifying moment, he severs the Dark Lord's head from his body. As the dark helmet falls to the ground, Luke watches in shocked disbelief as he stares down to see his own face looking up at him. Through this, Luke discovers that his greatest enemy is the fear, darkness, and evil lurking inside his own mind.

In stark contrast to the typical dark picture of the Inner Cave presented in the classic Hero's Journey, the Apostle Paul's words shine like a beacon of healing light and hope.

> *For we died and were buried with Christ by baptism. And just as Christ was raised from the dead by the glorious power of the Father, now we also may*

---

[142] Donald Gult, *Star Wars: The Empire Strikes Back Episode V* (New York: Random House Publishing Group, 1985), 148.

live new lives. Since we have been united with him in his death, we will also be raised to life as he was. We know that our old sinful selves were crucified with Christ so that sin might lose its power in our lives. We are no longer slaves to sin.
ROMANS 6:4-6 (NLT)

Unlike Luke Skywalker and the nebulous "force," we have a someone, not a something, who goes into the cave with us. Christ has already faced the ultimate Inner Cave—and his literal tomb—and emerged victorious. This gives you and I great confidence to walk boldly into our Inner Cave as well!

By now, you are probably asking yourself, *Why is the Hero's Journey so important for us to understand?* What Joseph Campbell discovered after studying hero stories from around the world for many years—and these stories were from a wide range of cultures—was that the heroes were all essentially taking the same journey. They would leave their ordinary lives and find themselves involved in an intense spiritual battle and, at times, it looked like the evil forces they were facing would crush them. But the forces of darkness are ultimately defeated; the Death Star explodes,[143] or as Joseph Campbell likes to say, "the dragon is slain."[144] In the process, the individual has changed from an average Joe to a hero.

But in order to see the ultimate defeat of evil, every hero must battle themselves and the old self—the darkness within. Luke Skywalker had to face the fear that he was destined to join the dark side. Frodo Baggins had to overcome the dark pull of the One Ring on his own mind. They both entered the cave of fear, but emerged stronger. Or, as Joseph Campbell himself puts it, "The cave you fear to enter holds the treasure you seek."[145] In facing this inner cave, we can emerge with greater confidence and clarity than ever before!

What fear are you battling with right now in your life?

---

[143] *Star Wars: Episode IV - A New Hope*, directed by George Lucas (San Francisco: Lucasfilm, 1977), film.

[144] *Joseph Campbell and the Power of Myth*, an interview with Bill Moyers (New York: Alvin H. Perlmutter, 1988), TV Mini Series.

[145] Diane K. Osbon, *Reflections on the Art of Living: A Joseph Campbell Companion* (New York: Harper Collins, 1991), 8, 24.

Which Fruit of the Spirit (Galatians 5:22-23) will you need in your life to release your warrior's heart?

___

Courage isn't a specific Fruit of the Spirit. Instead, it's a result of several Fruit of the Spirit brought to bear on the forces of hell in the spiritual battles we will encounter on the Hero's Journey. Hell will not be able to stand against us as we exhibit the Fruit of the Spirit. **When the Fruit of the Spirit flows through you, it will devastate hell!** For the simple reason that hell has no love, joy, peace, patience or self-control. Therefore you can truly ruin hell's plans when you walk in the Fruit of the Spirit!

A while ago, Diane and I decided to go back to a place with a lot of memories for us: Pensacola, Florida. This is the place where we were married and where I went through basic flight training. Just for fun, I went out on the running trails where I had spent hours of agony in strenuous physical activity.

I ended up standing beside a set of pull-up bars where, 40 years ago, they were a very significant part of my life. The year was 1968: the Vietnam War was in full swing and the Marine Corps was attempting to graduate as many pilots as quickly as possible. But the pipeline for pilot training was backed up for months, so I found myself in a class of potential Navy pilots going through ground school and physical conditioning. I understood what the drill instructors (or DIs) were doing—I was a Marine in a Navy class; therefore, they expected me to beat everyone else in the class, especially when it came to physical training. I would listen to the critical voice of the DI but I would not let him determine my perceived value. After having completed basic training and officers training in the Corps, I could run all day with a fully loaded pack, so the runs at Pensacola, Florida, were a "piece of cake." The Holy Spirit was helping me develop the Fruit of the Spirit of self-control. He was helping to develop my ability to deal with the voice of the critic within. Forty years later, I was standing there listening to a present-day DI challenging the group of officer candidates that he could do more pull-ups than they could ever do.

As I stood off to the side, the Lord brought to mind a scene from the movie, *An Officer and a Gentleman*.[146] Zack Mayo (played by Richard Gere) meets Sergeant Foley (played by Lou Gossett, Jr.) and the Sergeant believes Zack lacks motivation and is not a team player, which is a cardinal sin in the Corps. So Sergeant Foley begins to focus with sadistic intensity on the young candidate, trying to get him to DOR (drop on request). Zack refuses. Then Zack comes to a critical moment of total frustration and complete exhaustion. Zack finally admits the voice of Sergeant Foley is right; there are no options in civilian life for him. This understanding lays the foundation for Zack to acknowledge the reality of his selfishness and out of the pain of that personal revelation, he commits to becoming *an officer and a gentleman*.

Later in the film, Zack rides his motorcycle back to the training area after graduating. Still in his Dress White uniform, he pauses for a moment as he watches his former tormentor and mentor verbally attack a fresh batch of officer candidates. One young man, in particular, became the focus of Foley's wrath. Zack listens to the same speech in the same tone of viciousness that he had personally received a few weeks earlier. Ensign Zack Mayo looks at the camera with a knowing smile, turns, and rides off.

Life comes full circle at times, when we find ourselves standing in the same place we have been before—as I did that day, listening to the DI challenge a new class of potential flight officers. The question is: in the process, have we grown to become a better human being? Have we allowed God, through His Holy Spirit, to truly transform us? If not, life has a frustrating way of sending us around the same loop, again and again, until the lesson has transformed us and this phase of growth is complete.

> ❝ The truth I have seen in so many men's lives is: **how we deal with the voice of our inner critic in our life will determine whether we stay stuck in unhealthy patterns or we learn to soar in Christ!**[147]

Where have you found yourself experiencing life coming full circle at times? List the times where you had to take another lap in life and the times where you, like Zack, realized you had graduated.

---

[146] *An Officer and a Gentleman*, directed by Taylor Hackford (Culver City: Lorimar Film Entertainment, 1982), film.

[147] The reason standing beside those pull-up bars was so significant for me is, like Zack, I had heard the same speech they had heard from the DI. I took it as a challenge rather than as a put down. As a result, I set the pull-up record for the ground school.

ANOTHER LAP...	I GRADUATED!
Example: I masturbated again.	*Example: I have been free of porn and masturbation for a year!*
1.	1.
2.	2.
3.	3.
4.	4.
5.	5.

Hopefully, some items on your list will be areas of future graduation. For example, if you struggle with feeling defensive when having conflict with your wife, a future graduation would be: I didn't get defensive with my wife when I was upset.

You have probably put the pieces together by now. The overarching transforming circle that we can experience in our lives is about the eight stages of the Hero's Journey, which we looked at in the introduction. However, life can feel like we are living in a series of mini-circles at times, but the Holy Spirit is headed somewhere in our lives. Each mini-circle or loop within this lifelong journey brings our God-given calling into greater focus. The role of the hero is to serve and to sacrifice for others. The only guarantee we have is knowing we will be tested and challenged as every hero has been before us. So, tell hell to bring it on! This is so much better than sitting in your La-Z-Boy chair watching ESPN waiting for something exciting to happen.

A hero is ultimately someone who gives their life for something bigger than themselves. In essence, something deep inside is awakened within the hero, calling him to step forth from an ordinary life. **The hero's call is to change.** The God-given change is designed to wake up and shake up the man of God within.

The Inner Cave experience is a set up by God underlining the major conflict of the quest. We are approaching the deepest and darkest part of the journey. There are two things we must understand for this journey to grow into a transforming experience:

01. A growing sense of God's calling and purpose in our life. Or, as Joseph Campbell likes to put it, "Follow your Bliss!"[148]
02. Developing great skills when relating to our inner critic.

The frequent statements Campbell made about "following your bliss" initially sounded new age and a little fuzzy to me. Then I began to listen more carefully and realized he was speaking of God's call in a believer's life.

Now, by no stretch of the imagination do I believe Campbell understood what he was saying biblically. But at times, he could make comments freighted with such biblical insight, it was impressive. Such as his numerous observations about joy in life: "You should do that thing that fills you with the most joy and do it no matter what it is. That is the starting point of the real-life hero's journey."[149]

My story is a classic example of finding the God-given joy in life and pursuing it no matter what. I found myself feeling like I was "stuck" in life. I had accomplished my dream, I was a fighter pilot, but I sensed deep within that **something was missing**. In one of those incredible "it just happened" moments, the Holy Spirit revealed the reason why I was on this earth. My phone suddenly rang in the middle of the night. A doctor at the base hospital informed me that one of my Marines on the squadron's maintenance crew had attempted suicide. This act speaks of a horrific level of shame. Marines don't commit suicide; they cause the other side to commit suicide!

The medical staff had this guy isolated in the corner of the hospital. He was awash in shame. For the first time in my life, I deeply felt God's love for another human being. That night, I discovered the greatest joy for me was to help guys who were hurting, not just to fly fighter aircraft and land them on the aft end of a bouncing carrier.

To be honest, it took me several years before I would risk everything and begin the Hero's Journey of following my God-given joy.

Once again, Joseph Campbell eloquently expressed this truth:

> **Find a place inside where there's joy, and the joy will burn out the pain.**[150]

---

[148] Joseph Campbell, *The Power of Myth* (New York: Anchor Books, 1991), 113.

[149] *Joseph Campbell and the Power of Myth*, an interview with Bill Moyers (New York: Alvin H. Perlmutter, 1988), TV Mini Series.

[150] Joseph Campbell Quotes, BrainyQuote.com, BrainyMedia Inc, 2003. https://www.brainyquote.com/citation/quotes/joseph_campbell_384345.

Are you still caught in the crazy cycle of relapse no matter what you do? Or, are you experiencing sobriety but feel like you are a long way from living life to the fullest as Jesus promised? One of the possible answers to these frustrating dilemmas is discovering your God-given joy. Remember, sexual bondage at its core is about the self-destructive ways you have learned to medicate your pain within, which usually started in your childhood.

So where is your place of joy? What makes you feel alive?

Where do you need to take risks in your life to move toward your place of joy?

If you can't answer the first two questions in depth, then write a prayer expressing your desperate desire for God to reveal to you your place of joy in this hurting world.

Joseph Campbell declared that on our journey, there is a dragon we all must slay. He described the dragon as a beast covered with scales and on every scale is the declaration of either "Thou Shalt" or "Thou Shall Not."[151] After helping thousands of men come to health, I believe what Campbell is talking about is the critic within. He is talking about our deepest fears. Therefore, the Ordeal, the Inner Cave, is not about us getting rid of our worries but **confronting them**. Living life with courage is not about being fearless; it is about developing the character to face our fears—sometimes on a

---

[151] *Joseph Campbell and the Power of Myth*, an interview with Bill Moyers (New York: Alvin H. Perlmutter, 1988), TV Mini Series.

daily basis. The terms "Ordeal" and "the Inner Cave" speak metaphorically of life and death. Thus both metaphorically will kill you and make you stronger.

Everything that happens on the Hero's Journey leads up to this moment—the Ordeal. Everything afterward is about returning home. And there is no place like home![152] In Exodus, we find a classic story of a people dealing with an Ordeal and having to face their Inner Cave as Israel struggles to move into the promised land God had prepared for them.

> *"Now get yourselves ready. I'm sending my Angel ahead of you to guard you in your travels, to lead you to the place that I've prepared. Pay close attention to him. Obey him. Don't go against him. He won't put up with your rebellions because he's acting on my authority. But if you obey him and do everything I tell you, I'll be an enemy to your enemies; I'll fight those who fight you. When my Angel goes ahead of you and leads you to the land of the Amorites, the Hittites, the Perizzites, the Canaanites, the Hivites, and the Jebusites, I'll clear the country of them. So don't worship or serve their gods;…"*
>
> *"And I'll send Despair in ahead of you. It will push the Hivites, the Canaanites, and the Hittites out of your way. I won't get rid of them all at once lest the land grow up in weeds and the wild animals take over. Little by little, I'll get them out of there while you have a chance to get your crops going and make the land your own. I will make your borders stretch from the Red Sea to the Mediterranean Sea and from the Wilderness to the Euphrates River. I'm turning everyone living in that land over to you;…"*
>
> EXODUS 23:20-24, 28-31 (MSG)

There is a truth that stands out in Exodus 23, but it's not as much fun to look at. It's the phrase, "little by little." How long does it usually take a guy to not just stop acting out but to ultimately be free? Answer: two to five years, little by little.

This dynamic passage demonstrates how God can have angels protect you and bring you to the place, but the angel can't go in for you. Even God can set up everything, but He can't take the step for you. If God did this it wouldn't be kind; it would be cruel. He would be putting you in a place where your faith couldn't stand. The great tragedy in this passage is that an entire generation failed to enter into the Promised Land because they never dealt with the critic within. Numbers 13:33 describes how the Israelites saw themselves in comparison to the present occupants of the land: "…*we were like grasshoppers in our own sight*…" God brought them to their Inner Cave and they turned back in fear. How about you?

---

[152] As I write this chapter, I am sitting in a VA rehab center in Vancouver, Washington. I had a hip replacement surgery and my Parkinson's triggered, so they would not let me go home. When I wrote the statement, "There is no place like home," tears came to my eyes. Ordeals in our life can bring a depth of character and thankfulness that can happen no other way in our lives.

Dealing with your Inner Critic

For the majority of the next chapter, we will be learning exactly how to deal with the critic within, but first of all, we need to understand clearly what we mean by the term "inner critic." I would define the inner critic as **an internal voice that often produces negative feelings of shame, insignificance, worthlessness, low self-esteem, self-doubt, and a lack of self-confidence**. Nearly everyone struggles with an inner critic. For example, individuals who struggle with depression have severe inner critics and tend to engage in intense internal fights with the critical voice within. This means there are many types of critics we can find ourselves facing. For more information and understanding about the character of your inner critic, take the quiz found at: **https://personal-growth-programs.com/inner-critic-section**.

This analysis will help us change our perspective toward our inner critic. We need to develop the ability to step back from our inner critic and not be so afraid of it. We can easily become emotionally reactive toward our inner critic, but we need to build a sense of curiosity and compassion toward it. I know this is going to be a challenge for some of you; but remember, this is the doorway for many to stop the insane cycle of relapse in your life. As your inner critic becomes your companion, your weakness will be transformed into your strength by the grace of God.

So, let's close this chapter by taking some time before the Lord and thoughtfully answer these questions. Take your time and write out your answers. Use a separate sheet of paper if necessary.

When you think about your inner critic:

How does it sound?

_____
_____
_____
_____

Who does it sound like?

_____
_____
_____
_____

What is its job?

What are its greatest fears?

How old is it?

If you were to draw a picture or cartoon of it, how would it look?

Who is it trying to protect?

BE PREPARED TO SHARE WITH YOUR GROUP YOUR ANSWERS TO THE QUESTIONS IN THIS CHAPTER.

CHAPTER 14
THE EXILE WITHIN IS FINALLY HONORED

As we begin this week, take some time and reflect back on the Inner Critic quiz and the work you did in your group around this topic. Learning to recognize this voice is key to moving forward, so let's drill down a little deeper:

What did you find interesting about your results from the Inner Critic quiz?

_____
_____
_____
_____

What are the three most powerful critics in your life?

01. _____
02. _____
03. _____

What does this say about your past and your view of yourself? How long have you struggled with this voice in your head?

_____
_____
_____
_____
_____

Several years ago, as I wrestled with these questions, I finally realized why I had battled with relapse for so long in my life. It dawned on me that I was expecting sanctification to work in my life the same as salvation. They are both released in our lives through grace, God's grace! But there is a massive difference in experiencing forgiveness and walking in sustained freedom! Forgiveness is immediately ours in Christ, but sanctification involves a process. This is why freedom in certain areas of our life can take years.

There is an even more profound question that troubles the soul of the thoughtful reader who tries to understand the severe emotional contrasts we can find in Scripture. The classic example is the jarring dissonance between Romans 6 and 7. Paul speaks with such passion and joy of our freedom in Christ in Romans 6, but then he radically changes focus in Romans 7. He is suddenly speaking from the depths of personal despair and frustration.

> *But I need something more! For if I know the law but still can't keep it, and if the power of sin within me keeps sabotaging my best intentions, I obviously need help! I realize that I don't have what it takes. I can will it, but I can't do it. I decide to do good, but I don't really do it; I decide not to do bad, but then I do it anyway. My decisions, such as they are, don't result in actions. Something has gone wrong deep within me and gets the better of me every time.*
>
> ROMANS 7:18-20 (MSG)

Some would say Paul is talking about past struggles in his life; this may be true in verses 7-13, where Paul's words are framed in his past: "I was," or "I would not." Here he is describing in painful detail the battle he discovered he could never win. In verses 14-25, however, he shifts entirely to the present tense: "I am," "I do," and "I know." He begins to delineate the battle we must choose to never lose!

If you're married, and as a couple, you have probably figured out it is not an easy process to walk in the freedom Christ purchased for you on Calvary's Cross. And if you are single, it is also tricky. The reason for this is: the very thing we hunger for the most is also the very thing we tend to fear the most. We all deeply crave intimacy—to be fully known and accepted. But it is usually the fear of intimacy that causes us to withdraw because of wounds from our past. This is why I frequently say to the men gathered at a conference, "Gentlemen, the way you love your wife is the way you love Christ! Don't cut it any other way because I have never met a man who is close to God and isn't close to his wife as well."

So what is the answer to the intense conflict between Romans 6 and 7? Some would say the answer is simply found in Romans 8. However, this chapter is the longest of the entire complex argumentation of Romans. Therefore, the answer is not so obvious. But if we read Romans 8 carefully, it offers a fascinating insight into the **process** of sanctification which can help us understand how to experience real freedom in our lives.

All around us we observe a pregnant creation. The difficult times of pain throughout the world are simply birth pangs. But it's not only around us; it's within us. The Spirit of God is arousing us within. We're also feeling the birth pangs. These sterile and barren bodies of ours are yearning for full deliverance. That is why waiting does not diminish us, any more than waiting diminishes a pregnant mother. We are enlarged in the waiting.

ROMANS 8:22-25 (MSG)

Paul uses the incredible example of a woman giving birth to a child. He is underlining the fact that it is never instantaneous. If it is a healthy birth, the **process** takes approximately nine months. I have seen so many men caught in the insane cycle of relapse but this is an insane cycle of spiritual miscarriage; they are expecting to check all the boxes in the *Seven Pillars of Freedom* curriculum and Shazam!—they will be free. I always remember what Dr. Carnes said to me: "It takes at least two to five years for a sex addict to come to health." I have found this to be so true! For Christ-followers, however, I have made a significant adjustment to Dr. Carnes statement: "It can take only one to three years for a man who walks with Christ into the freedom He purchased for him on the Cross. The process may be reduced slightly but will need a miracle every day for this to occur."

What is the essence of this process and where does it primarily take place? Paul makes it crystal clear in Romans 12.

And do not be conformed to this world [any longer with its superficial values and customs], but be transformed and progressively changed [as you mature spiritually] by the renewing of your mind [focusing on godly values and ethical attitudes], so that you may prove [for yourselves] what the will of God is, that which is good and acceptable and perfect [in His plan and purpose for you].

ROMANS 12:2 (AMP)

The **process** of renewing our mind which Paul is referring to is not some data download we acquire in a discipleship program. Instead, it involves "proving for ourselves what the will of God is for our lives." He is talking about new experiences, not just more information. Therefore, he is not talking about building up our higher reasoning processes by providing new input to our prefrontal cortex. The renewing of our mind which Paul is referring to takes place at the limbic level. It is a subconscious process. And the limbic system (which deals specifically with your will and emotions) is only transformed toward health as we encounter **new, positive experiences that are directly counter to deeply wounding traumatic experiences of our past**.

This is precisely why the healing process can take so long. There is no way we can quickly deal with family of origin issues. We also can't instantly deal with traumatic moments that shaped our lives and our view of reality. The Arousal Template, which lies at the core of why we do what we don't want to do, will not give up its secrets effortlessly. Three areas of significant wounding in a man's soul need to be purposefully addressed in their life if there is any hope of real healing:

01. Family of origin issues (Pillars 1-4, *Seven Pillars of Freedom*)

02. The Arousal Template (Pillar 5, *Seven Pillars of Freedom*)

03. Traumatic moments from the past (Pillar 6, *Seven Pillars of Freedom*)

Now the thing that makes this whole process so challenging is, the areas of wounding are at the subconscious level. Therefore the enemy's attacks are usually in stealth mode. We don't even realize we are wounded. We end up living in a fake world we don't fully understand.

It's a little bit like *The Truman Show*,[153] in which Jim Carrey plays a man who is living in a fake world. In fact, the place he lives is a big studio with hidden cameras everywhere; all his friends and people around him are actors who play their roles in the most popular TV series in the world. In the movie, an interviewer once asked Christof, the creator of this wildly popular reality show, why Truman never realized he lived in a false world. The satanic creator slyly smiled and said, "**We accept the reality of the world with which we're presented; it's as simple as that.**"[154]

The reason I labeled Christof as being satanic is because the most potent weapon he used against Truman was fear. When Truman was a small child, Christof staged the death of his father in a mock sailing accident in the bay. Ever since then, Truman has been terrified of the water, which keeps him confined to the island so that the show can continue.

At times, the truth that Truman dealt with didn't make any sense. In the opening scene of the movie, a stage light falls from the sky and crashes to the ground. As Truman is driving to work, he hears a news flash over the radio announcing that an aircraft flying over Seahaven had lost some parts. But stage lights are not designed to be part of an airplane.

Truman's hunger for the truth is far more than just a passing interest. Another character in the movie, Sylvia, was an actress with a script to follow like everyone else. One problem: she fell in love with Truman. Sylvia soon realized her days were numbered once her acting departed from the required text. Before they yanked her from the show, she quickly tries to explain to Truman the pseudo nature of the world he finds himself trapped in and how he's the real character of a show the world is watching. As she leaves, Sylvia manages to break through all the falsehoods of the TV show and looks deeply into Truman's eyes, expressing a heartfelt challenge to him: "Come and find me!"[155]

---

[153] *The Truman Show*, directed by Peter Weir (Hollywood: Paramount Pictures, 1998), film.

[154] *The Truman Show*.

[155] *The Truman Show*.

With Sylvia removed from his life, he realizes that the answers to his most profound questions can only be discovered by sailing boldly into his fear. He knows, somehow, the truth would become real to him as he faced his fears; so he sets sail. Christof unleashes a storm on Truman, certain his fears will overpower him. But Truman fastens himself to the boat with his body in cruciform and cries out against the wind and waves, "Is that the best you can do? You are going to have to kill me!"[156] He wants the truth so badly, he is willing to die for it!

After the storm has subsided, the pivotal moment of freedom comes when Truman fights back the tears, reaches out, and cautiously touches the wall. Suddenly, the truth becomes crystal clear: everything behind him was a lie. Christof, his demonic adversary, created all his fears. Truman sees a door marked "Exit" but for a second, he ponders his options. Everything behind him was familiar but false. Everything on the other side of the door is unknown. Truman takes a final bow to the TV audience and walks through the door. Sylvia, who has been waiting on the other side, runs to embrace him!

I teared up when I watched Truman walk through the exit because it reminded me of so many men I have walked with through the year-long counseling process. As we begin the process, there is nothing but hostility between him and his wife. But slowly, he starts to realize how ill-equipped he is to resolve marital conflicts. His father had never loved his mother because of the deep dysfunctions that existed in their home. He had never learned how to genuinely love a woman. His wife, whom he has severely betrayed, has hung in there with him. Once he finally faces his fears and wakes up to the falsehood he has lived in, he finally realizes what an incredible gift his wife is to him. However, this realization and healing process takes at least a year, which brings us back to Exodus 23, which we looked at in the last chapter. In verse 28, we find another fascinating statement:

> *I will send the hornet ahead of you to drive the Hivites, Canaanites and Hittites out of your way. But I will not drive them out in a single year, because the land would become desolate and the wild animals too numerous for you. Little by little I will drive them out before you, until you have increased enough to take possession of the land.*
>
> EXODUS 23:28-30 (NIV)

There is no agreement among biblical scholars what "the hornet or wasp" is referring to, but in the previous verse, it is clear what is taking place. Their enemies are terrified and running for cover! Sadly, the Israelites ended up running from an enemy that God had already defeated. They didn't understand how, at times, **the devil's tools of torment can become God's tools of transformation**. Israel's enemy will be driven from the land, BUT it would not be instantaneously. Meaning they would need to deal with the hornets and wild animals as well.

---

[156] *The Truman Show.*

I finally got it! Now I understand why God left the giants in the Promised Land. He had subcontracted them! So, you don't need to worry about the enemy you may be presently facing. The Lord declares, "They are working for me!"

Recently, as I violently struggled with Parkinson's disease, I cried out for God to take this weakness away. He quietly whispered to my soul, "No, Ted, I am going to work through it. Your weakness will force you to depend on Me. It will lead you to My strength." At that moment, I realized how much of my identity had been built on my physical abilities as a college gymnastics, fighter pilot, and triathlete. I didn't know who I was apart from my physical skills; all my life, my inner critic had driven me to prove myself. Since I was a child, I had lived with this haunting voice within telling me I wasn't good enough. Since I had a parade of stepfathers walk through my life who never had time for me, it's easy to see how I came to live with such a nagging inner critic.

If you grew up with a disinterested, perfectionist, or emotionally absent father you will probably suffer from a sense of uncertainty as to who you are. You will experience confusion about your worth and your special uniqueness. Most of the men I have counseled who did not have a positive father's voice in their lives spent most of their life looking for themselves in all the wrong places.

What five adjectives would you use to describe your father?

01. _____
02. _____
03. _____
04. _____
05. _____

The amazing fact in all of this is, sometimes, God will use the devil to deliver His mail. God took what the enemy had tried to torment me with and used it to transform me. Through Exodus 23, I learned how to thank God, not just for His protection, but for the giants I had to face as well. It was in facing my fears of Parkinson's disease where I discovered who I truly am.

Danny Gokey's hit song, *Tell Your Heart To Beat Again*,[157] has become my Inner Cave battle cry.

---

[157] Danny Gokey, "Tell Your Heart to Beat Again." Track 3 on *Hope in Front of Me*. GMB Rights Management, 2016, CD.

You're shattered
Like you've never been before
The life you knew
In a thousand pieces on the floor
And words fall short in times like these
When this world drives you to your knees
You think you're never gonna get back
To the you that used to be…

Love's healing hands have pulled you through
So get back up, take step one…
'Cause your story's far from over
And your journey's just begun

Tell your heart to beat again…

In meeting the giants, I learned how to fight; they built my faith. I have learned new compassion for disabled folks. I have let go of my arrogance and I'm learning a new humility.

It is one thing to praise God for His protection, but it is another level of trust to thank Him for your problems. Sometimes your problems are God's protection from yourself.

What are the problems in your life—the giants God is using in your life right now to heal you and grow you up?

_____
_____
_____
_____
_____
_____

Write a prayer thanking God for the blessings you've experienced while facing the problems in your life.

_____
_____
_____
_____
_____
_____

The previous quiz and questions concerning your inner critic come from a type of therapy known as Internal Family Systems Therapy (IFS).[158] Now relax, I am not going to drop a lot of psychobabble on you. In some ways, it is an intuitive approach and, amazingly enough, fits beautifully within a positive, Christ-centered approach. IFS therapy helps us see that we are all made up of "parts" or different aspects of ourselves. We have "exiles" who carry our pain, "managers" who cope with the pain or cover it (like a performer, or our inner critic), and "firefighters" who cope by putting out the pain when it really flares up (like our addiction).

Now Internal Family Systems can become a very complicated process when you are dealing with deeply traumatizing issues from your past.[159] However, I have found it very helpful for men who are struggling with sexual bondages in their lives, to give them some basic tools in dealing with their inner critic. So let's take on the giant critical voice in your head, like the Israelites, that keeps saying you're worthless, nothing but a grasshopper. From Exodus 23, we understand how God is using the inner critic's voice to get our attention about healing that needs to take place inside of us and to bring a greater sense of balance within our various parts. Otherwise, we will end up stuck in Romans 7, not understanding why we do what we don't want to do. We may assume we can deal with the giants like the Israelites did and get rid of them! However, there is a massive problem with this approach: the inner critic is part of us. This is why we usually can't win an argument with our inner critic and why we can't banish his voice for long.

This is also why the final question I asked you in Chapter 13 is so important: "Who is it trying to protect?" The inner critic's intent is usually positive, even if you don't appreciate its effect. Initially, this can be somewhat confusing because of the pain the inner critic is trying to prevent. The critic is often causing far more pain through his efforts to protect the child—or the exile—within. The critic is stuck in the past. As a child, there once was a real danger or harm that could hurt you. The critic doesn't realize you are now an adult and have many more options and capabilities to protect yourself.

When I am helping a client realize the crippling pain they suffered in their family of origin, I start by asking them if the inner critic's voice in their head sounds familiar. They will usually blurt out, "Yes, it sounds just like Mom..." or their dad or another family member. And frequently they will feel guilty for such an unguarded statement. To which I respond, "We are not blaming your mom or dad or family. They did the best they could with what they had."

---

[158] Richard C. Schwartz, *Internal Family Systems Therapy* (New York: The Guilford Press, 1995).

[159] The suggestions I have given you in this chapter will only be helpful if you are not dealing with any **significant** past traumatizing events. Therefore, if you find the suggestions frustrating or triggering a strong reaction within, please contact https://selfleadership.org/find-an-ifs-therapist.html online and they will help you find a certified IFS counselor.

So frequently, the inner critic's voice is simply an echo from the past still treating you like a child, ignoring the fact that you are now a responsible adult. Paul repeats a command that appears often in Scripture and then makes an interesting observation in Ephesians 6.

> *"For the commandment, 'Honor your father and your mother,' was the first of the Ten Commandments with a promise attached: 'You will prosper and live a long, full life if you honor your parents."*
> EPHESIANS 6:2-3 (TPT)

Is Paul saying, "Mom and Dad are always right; if you disagree with them, your life will be cut short?" Unfortunately, if you grew up in a dysfunctional religious home, this was the message that was drilled into you. The result is Mom and Dad ended up replacing God on the throne of your life. Remember, He is the only one who is always right. With this kind of thinking, you transform a generational blessing with a generational curse. Paul was emphasizing how your family of origin will have a significant impact on the way you look at and process life. It's important to realize the generational patterns that can be controlling your life and how often you are not even aware of it! Consider a past like mine: where there was total chaos, alcohol, and violence. A generational curse was part of the air I breathed even though I knew my mom loved me. The crazy thing is, at times, I can't seem to get her critical voice out of my head!

The question becomes, how do you counter this thinking and begin to walk to health?

First, recognize the pattern and become curious about your inner critic. How could my mom, who loved me so profoundly, become such a point of pain in my life? She must have experienced the generational curse in her life as well. This is why it is so important to be familiar with your inner critic's family background. Mom didn't share much about her early childhood, except for one comment she made about her mom. We were looking at some family pictures and I asked if she had any of her family. "Only one," she replied. I will never forget the image. In the picture, a little girl is standing beside an older woman. I asked her why the older lady looked so mad? Mom poignantly commented, "My mom never seemed to like me much; in fact, she threw me down a well and just left me there."

I was in grade school when she shared this with me so I didn't understand the severity of her comment. But after all the clinical training I've received, that simple statement my mom made helped me understand the voice of my inner critic. The world my mom grew up in was not a safe place; so she believed if she ever stopped trying to control my behavior, I would get hurt or in trouble. Of course, the high school years where I forged her signature to keep skydiving didn't help her feel safe about my crazy activities!

Is there the voice of a family member in your head? Chances are it has been there for more than one generation. What occurred in their past that would help you understand them and not be so triggered by them?

Second, recognize the connection between the exile and the inner critic. Here is where your story can become very interesting. Whenever an inner critic is active, there are actually two parts involved.[160] In addition to the critic, there is the exile or criticized child within. The exile is usually a younger part of you tied to a painful moment in your past. The exile is frozen in time because something difficult or traumatic happened then and you didn't have the inner resources or support to handle it. Therefore, you were overwhelmed and couldn't process what was happening. This part of you is stuck there!

The inner critic is judging or criticizing the exile and as a result, the child within is feeling shame or feeling bad about themselves. Essentially, the inner critic is telling the criticized child how to behave or not behave. The inner critic has a very frustrating job; they don't have the power to act in the world directly. Their judgments are derived from the difficulty of getting the child to act in a way they feel would protect them. In reality, most inner critics are parts that developed their protective strategy when they were young, reflecting the family of origin. Thus, they lack the capacity to act in mature ways and they don't realize the child now has abilities and resources they never had in their family of origin.

As an adult who loves Christ, you now have an adult brain with a fully developed prefrontal cortex that is able to problem-solve and logically think things through. You also have the Holy Spirit working within you and your Pure Desire group members can affirm and speak of God's healing grace over you. These are resources you never had in your family of origin.

---

[160] Actually your inner relational structure is much more complex than just these two parts but this is a great place to start understanding your Internal Family System. An excellent workbook to continue your personal investigation is: Frank Anderson, Martha Sweezy, and Richard Schwartz, *Internal Family Systems Skills Training Manual: Trauma-Informed Treatment for Anxiety, Depression, PTSD & Substance Abuse* (Eau Claire: PESI Publishing & Media, 2017).

The painful part is when the "exile" or criticized child accepts the rules of his dysfunctional family of origin and tries to live by them no matter how debilitating or harmful they may be. So many times, I have had to challenge the rules a client grew up with because they were destroying him and his marriage. He was unknowingly recreating the sickness of his family of origin in his own family because it's what he was used to.

Finally, we need to free the inner critic from the role of protecting us. The ultimate goal is to heal all our parts and free them from the extreme roles they may have taken on because of the pain of the past. Then under the leadership of the Holy Spirit, to have your true self—your God-given nature—help them cooperate with each other. In the limited space we have in this chapter, we can't accomplish all of this; but what we can do is get to know our criticized child—or exile—within.

If you find these questions too triggering, please refer to footnote 158.

In a quiet space, take some deep, slow breaths. Become aware of your body and your thoughts. Don't try to force anything. Just relax and listen to whatever responses come to mind as you walk through this exercise. Ask the exile or child within:

How old are you?

What happened in your childhood that made you feel the way you do about yourself?

What feelings and beliefs do you have toward yourself?

How do you feel toward the child within or the exile?

What burdens or wounds is the child within carrying?

How would you like to release those burdens?

- ☐ Throw them into the sea?
- ☐ Have the fire of the Holy Spirit burn them up?
- ☐ Have the wind of the Holy Spirit blown them away?

Whichever option you selected, write down how you picture it happening.

Let me close by reminding you of the incident that took place in my life at Dr. Grand's Brainspotting Class, when I asked the Holy Spirit to open my eyes to what was happening beneath the surface of my life in dealing with my inner critic.[161]

The Holy Spirit used Dr. Grand's words that day to profoundly bring healing to my soul. This man, who I consider a father figure, had heard the story of my desire as a 5 year old to be a fighter pilot, and had looked deeply at me and said, "That is a fantastic kid, isn't he?" For the first time, Dr. Grand's voice totally silenced my inner critic voice, which had constantly told me I was never good enough. After a childhood filled with rejection by seven stepfathers and years as an alcoholic, sex addict, and rage-aholic, on top of all of the hell of Vietnam, my critic had an infinite number of things he could charge me with. These were the glasses hell had put over my eyes to see myself. Suddenly, Dr. Grand's question had opened my eyes to see a kid who had a heart for God right from the beginning! I was five and I had a heart for adventure! I had never seen myself this way before! The exile was finally honored—he was coming home to Father God!

God has a similar revelation for you to discover. Think about how your heavenly Father wants to welcome home the exile in your life. What might this look like for you?

_____
_____
_____
_____
_____
_____

Based on what you've learned so far, how is it helping you become a Compassionate Warrior? Be specific in your answer.

_____
_____
_____
_____
_____
_____

BE PREPARED TO SHARE WITH YOUR GROUP YOUR ANSWERS TO THE QUESTIONS IN THIS CHAPTER.

---

[161] David Grand, Master Brainspotting Class, Boulder, Colorado, 2013.

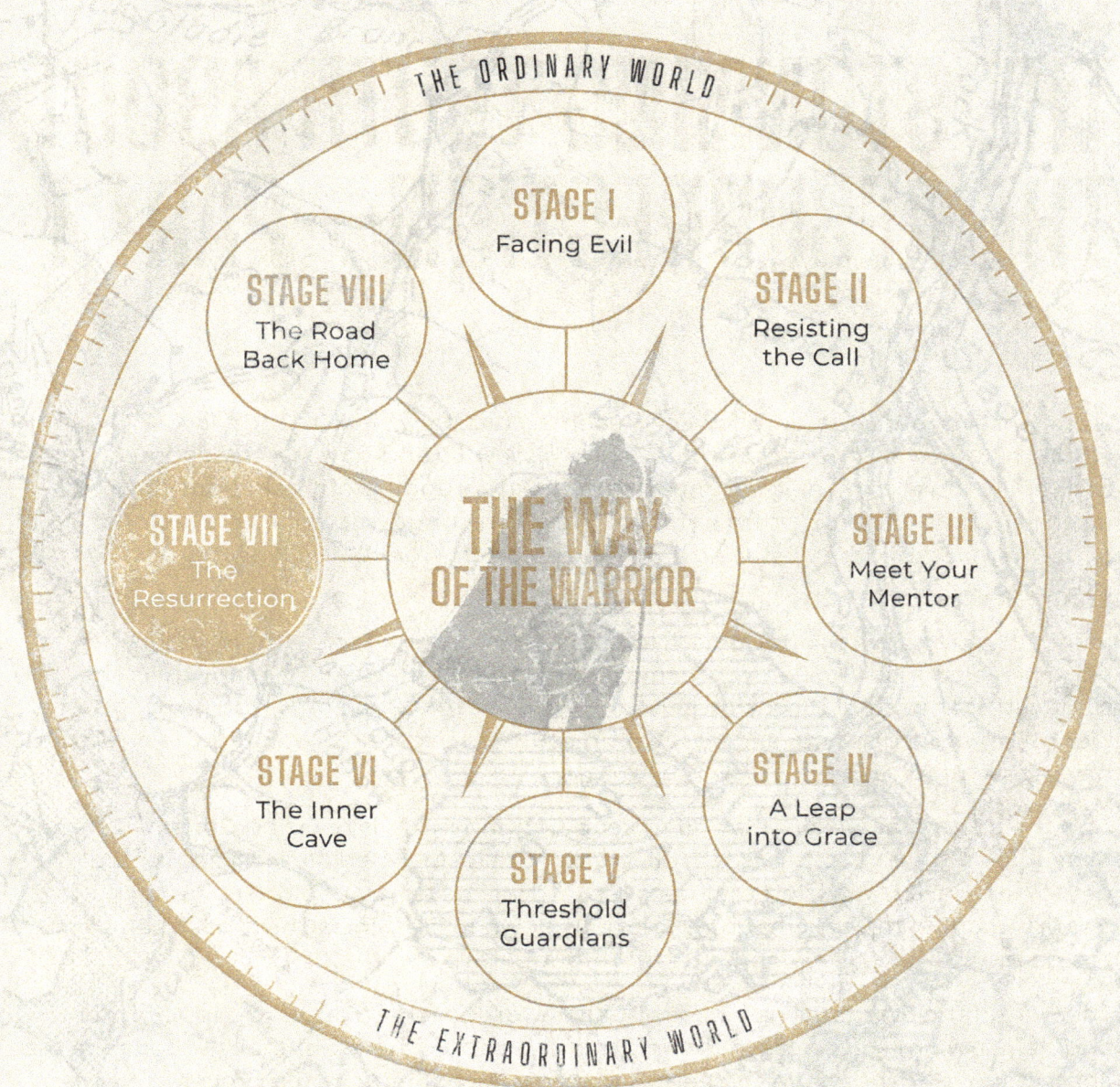

STAGE VII

THE RESURRECTION

CHAPTER 15
THE STUNNING TRUTH ABOUT THE RESURRECTION—PART 1

Have you ever noticed how a few folks seem to naturally walk in God's favor? My all-time favorite is *Forrest Gump*.[162] Despite his low IQ and physical restrictions, he literally runs from one encounter to the next, shrugging off limitations and discrimination. Life didn't turn out ideally for Forrest but when does it ever for any of us? Remarkably, the obstacles didn't keep Forrest from being kind, honest, and courageous.

In fact, I submit to you, our God is a lot like Forrest Gump. For example, when did Forrest ever stop loving Jenny? He never did! It didn't matter how many guys she slept with or how much cocaine she snorted. *Forrest loved Jenny*. (You need to say "Jenn-ay" with a distinctive Forrest Gump southern accent to get it right.) Forrest never gave up on Jenny!

And the thing that will enable you to keep fighting in life is realizing Christ will never give up on you—EVER. This is what living out the resurrected life is all about until we get to heaven. It is realizing that because God will never give up on us, we can always get up again no matter what may knock us down in life! Since Christ has risen from the dead, we also will overcome death through Him!

The Way of the Warrior is never easy but it is worth every struggle, disappointment, and defeat we may face. It's in the midst of the battle where we finally experience the character of Christ that we so deeply hunger for in our lives. In the process, relapse becomes something we no longer fear. **Instead, it becomes a learning experience where we discover God's grace and purpose for us because we don't allow shame to define us.** This is precisely why we don't have to repeat the insane cycle of shame and relapse, medicate the pain by acting out again, only to experience further shame.

Instead, we personally experienced the reality that God will never give up on us so we never give up on ourselves either. Over time, this process of never giving up on ourselves develops the character of Christ deep within us—but it is never an easy process!

---

[162] *Forrest Gump*, directed by Robert Zemeckis (Hollywood: Paramount Pictures, 1994), film.

> *Character cannot be developed in ease and quiet. Only through experience of trial and suffering can the soul be strengthened, ambition inspired and success achieved.*[163]
>
> HELEN KELLER

The Death and Resurrection of Christ is for us, both as an example of how the Resurrection changes us and also a new power to face areas in our own life where Death and Resurrection is needed. In 1 Corinthians 15, Paul makes clear the absolute priority of the Resurrection to our faith.

> *"But if there is no resurrection of the dead, then Christ is not risen. And if Christ is not risen, then our preaching is empty and your faith is also empty."*
>
> 1 CORINTHIANS 15:13-14 (NKJV)

Paul is dynamically illustrating how all of us are headed for a showdown moment at some point in our lives. A showdown is where we will be pitted against our greatest adversary and, in the process, the reality of the Resurrection will be demonstrated in our life.

In one of my all-time favorite "buddy" movies, *Butch Cassidy and the Sundance Kid*,[164] Butch and Sundance are surrounded and outnumbered. They respond by choosing to run head first into a wall of hostile gunfire. It is rather apparent they are about to die, but they decided to go down fighting! This freeze-frame moment has stuck in my memory unabated through the years. Paul's words in 1 Corinthians 15, however, have created a far more significant freeze-frame moment in my mind and it's more impactful than any Hollywood movie. Church tradition tells us that the apostle was beheaded, probably by a military execution squad with a sword. The executioner was commonly one of the Praetorian bodyguards for such a significant political prisoner; and the act was performed in the presence of a centurion, whose duty was to see the sentence carried out. In Philippians 1:12-14, we find the fascinating comment about how Paul's imprisonment contributed to the advancement of the good news among all the Praetorian Guard.

> *I want to report to you, friends, that my imprisonment here has had the opposite of its intended effect. Instead of being squelched, the Message has actually prospered. All the soldiers here, and everyone else, too, found out that I'm in jail because of this Messiah. That piqued their curiosity, and now they've learned all about him. Not only that, but most of the followers of Jesus here have become far more sure of themselves in the faith than ever, speaking out fearlessly about God, about the Messiah.*
>
> PHILIPPIANS 1:12-14 (MSG)

---

[163] Helen Keller Quote, BrainyQuote, https://www.brainyquote.com/quotes/helen_keller_101340.

[164] *Butch Cassidy and the Sundance Kid*, directed by George Roy Hill (Hopkinsville: Campanile Productions, 1969), film.

The preaching wasn't empty. The power of Christ's Resurrection was so real and impactful, it turned the very people who directly or indirectly had executed him into some of the faith's most influential spokesmen of that day!

This Stage is all about YOU personally experiencing the Resurrection in your own life. As a student, you may have crammed for a final exam and done very well on the test. But the ultimate field test always awaits you, where your heart is radically tested in the real world. The actual life test I am referring to is the challenge you will face through your death in Christ. Your belief in Christ's sacrifice for you will become evident because of the significant changes in your life.

In the movie, *Witness*,[165] we find a vivid illustration of this truth: a cop comes to the final showdown with his most despised enemy, a crooked cop. The Amish people of his adopted community are watching closely to see if the policeman, John Book, will relapse back into the violent ways of the world or if he will follow the peaceful way. John has to make an agonizing choice between engaging in the inevitable gunfight or walking away from his old ways of dealing with intense conflict. He decides to put down his gun, which is a dangerous choice and, instead, he stands with the silent Amish. Like them, he is a witness, thus the title of the movie. The "old man" John Book wouldn't think twice about a shoot-out with his enemy. He would have just pulled the trigger. The "new man" chose not to pull the trigger.

I remember sitting with several guys in a classic Pure Desire group meeting. One gentleman was complaining about how his fifteen-year-old son's disrespect had triggered his anger. What he didn't realize is that he was struggling with an encounter moment of the most important kind: a father versus son moment.

In his frustration he explained, "I tried everything you have told me to do. Just before I went ballistic with my son, I even asked myself, 'What am I afraid of?'"

"And what did you discover?" I inquired.

"I wasn't afraid of anything!" he almost shouted at me. "I can't allow my son to disrespect the **position** of me being his dad."

I paused for a long time, so the word "position" could hang in the air for all of us to evaluate its impact.

Instead of asking what the word "position" meant to him, I reviewed some facts I had found to be true among the men I had counseled. I asked them, for probably the one-hundredth time, "How many of you are struggling with a deep father wound?" They all raised their hands. I told them this was true for over 80% of the men I had worked with who struggle with sexual bondage. Then I added how over 90% of those men had an angry dad and he had mentored them well!

---

[165] *Witness*, directed by Peter Weir (Hollywood: Paramount Pictures, 1985), film.

Being raised by an angry, distant, or uncaring dad will trigger deep insecurities in your soul. And this is what so frequently drives your angry limbic responses toward your sons.

I circled back around and asked the fear question once again, "So what were you afraid of?" He responded, "I guess, I was afraid my son's disrespect toward me would make me look bad."

"Exactly!" I shouted for joy; "And this is why you became so focused on your **position**." I went on to explain how his anger wasn't really about his son; instead, it was a reaction driven by the fear of not being a good dad, or husband, or…fill in the blank. He was unconsciously treating his son the way his dad had treated him. He was communicating in anger to his son the way his dad had spoken to him.

After he shared his angry response to his son, I smiled and asked my perennial "Dr. T" question: "How's that working for you?" He quickly caught the intent of my comment because he sensed my heart for him. He smiled in return and expressed how his deep father wound is an area that still needs some work. This is the test that proves he has learned a critical lesson in life; and he is a new man, a resurrected man!

As Paul put it, if you have not experienced the Resurrection touch of God in your life, then your faith lacks substance.

> So in your family or your community, where do those closest to you need to see change? Is it in your anger or your tendency to control; or the other extreme, to avoid confrontation and become passive?

> Where does your family need to see you stand as a witness for Christ? Where do they need to see the Resurrection power of God at work in your life? If you are not sure, ask them and add their responses to your own answers.

In the next chapter, we will look at what God would challenge you to do with such information and what He is calling you to change and ultimately become in your life.

For now, let's take a deep dive into how this Resurrection power produces change in us and in future generations—all the way down to our cells!

The concept of generational curses first appears in Exodus 20:5. In the King James Version, it says that God will "visit" the sins of the fathers down to the third and fourth generation. The term "visit" makes more sense in light of recent studies, which show that generational curses can, indeed, be scientifically traced back from one generation to another. But on a personal note, this explains why some patterns in our family history seem to be recurring in our life, like our dad's anger.

> List some patterns you have wrestled with from your family history. Is it the way your family tends to deal with relational struggles? Some other examples of negative family history being passed along are anger, perfectionism, judgmental attitudes, trying to control others, or my family's favorite—denial of any and all emotions! What are yours?

01. _____

02. _____

03. _____

The types of scientific studies of families are "longitudinal" studies which is a term used to describe an observational research method where data is gathered from the same subjects repeatedly over time. Through such research, they have discovered that alcoholism, drug addiction, anxiety, and even poverty can be recurring patterns in specific families.[166]

Let's set theology aside for a moment; common sense tells us that behavior and attitude problems—just like physical characteristics of height, weight, hair color, and complexion—tend to run in families. In the same way, certain types of sin flow from generation to generation—addictive behaviors such as alcoholism or sexual addiction. Similarly, physical and sexual abuse might become ingrained in the psychological legacy of particular families. But does it mean we should view our struggles with alcoholism or sexual addiction as an irreversible "curse?" Does DNA doom us and dictate that such battles flow from parents or grandparents and come down to us? Are we simply a product of our genes? NO!

Romans 10:13 declares that spiritual deliverance is available to everyone who sincerely calls upon the name of the Lord.

---

[166] Jack P. Shonkoff and Samuel J. Meisels, *Handbook of Early Childhood Intervention*, 2nd ed. (Cambridge: Cambridge University Press, 2000), 116.

And it's true: "Everyone who calls on the Lord's name will experience new life."
ROMANS 10:13 (TPT)

The only qualification for you to experience a new life is through sincerely calling on the Lord. Now you might ask the question, "So how do we change something science tells us is unchangeable?" The joyous good news from Romans 10:13 was astutely proclaimed six hundred years before the birth of Christ by the Old Testament prophet, Jeremiah, in anticipation of His coming.

"In those days people will no longer say, 'The parents have eaten sour grapes. But the children have a bitter taste in their mouths.' Instead, everyone will die for their own sin. The one who eats sour grapes will taste how bitter they are."
JEREMIAH 31:29-30 (NIRV)

Jeremiah realized God was going to change things so dramatically through the coming Messiah and every individual would be responsible for their own choices. The Messiah could set us free from the twisted entanglements and fatalism of generational curses. In the end, the only choice that counts is how we answer the ultimate question in life: "What shall I do with Jesus, who is called the Christ?"

Modern scientific studies have recently caught up with this biblical revelation. Pioneering research in the field of epigenetics reveals that our life experiences and choices change us; including our brains, down to the DNA level.[167] Therefore, our genes are not our destiny! And these changes can be passed onto our children to the fourth generation through our diet, work environment, and all of our significant choices. They can change the genetic legacy we pass on to our children and grandchildren.

The term "epigenetics" is from two words. First, the Greek word "epi" which means around or over the gene; and second, the word "genetics" which refers to the study of the cell's DNA.[168] The proteins which surround the DNA can cause specific genes to turn on and others to remain dormant. These changes in gene activity may stay for the remainder of the cell's life and may also last for three to four generations of cells. However, there is no change in the underlying DNA sequence of the organism. The fact that there is no change didn't seem possible only a few years ago.

---

[167] National Scientific Council on the Developing Child, *Early Experiences Can Alter Gene Expression and Affect Long-Term Development: Working Paper No. 10*. May 2010, http://www.developingchild.net.

[168] Nessa Carey, *The Epigenetics Revolution: How Modern Biology is Rewriting Our Understanding of Genetics, Disease, and Inheritance* (New York: Columbia University Press, 2012), 7-8.

In 2007, Dr. Randy Jirtle, professor at Duke University, gravely shook up the scientific community when he uncovered the reality of epigenetics.[169] Let me cut through all the biological terminology by using an analogy Nessa Carey used in his excellent introduction to the subject, *The Epigenetics Revolution*.[170] The cells would be the actors and actresses; the essential units that make up the movie. DNA, in turn, would be the script: instructions for all the participants of the film to perform their roles. The concept of epigenetics, then, would be like directing. The text can be the same but the director can choose to eliminate or tweak certain scenes or dialogue, altering the movie for better or worse. After all, Steven Spielberg's finished product would be drastically different from Woody Allen's rendition for the same movie script.

What's fascinating about this new area of scientific research is that it reveals how our DNA is not immutable, which was the former notion. Still, the environment clearly affects our gene expressions and the ways we function and behave. Thus, not only do we pass along the DNA sequence to our children but we also pass along the epigenetic instructions for them. In other words, information can be inherited and transmitted through generations. Science is simply confirming the truth of Scripture!

A perfect example of this is the effect of the 9/11 attacks.[171] Among the thousands of people directly exposed to the terrorist attack were 1,700 pregnant women. Some of these women developed symptoms of post-traumatic stress disorder (PTSD). They discovered their children reacted with high levels of fear and stress around loud noises, unfamiliar people, or new foods. It seems the infants inherited the nightmare their mothers experienced on that day.

Recent research also helps us understand why infants can be so affected by their mother's traumatic experiences. The pregnant mother's womb will have elevated levels of cortisol if she is exposed to high levels of stress. The mother's bloodstream prior to birth is essentially united with the child. Therefore, the child's basic setting for decisions about whether to fight, flight, or freeze in high stress situations were in some sense preprogrammed by the mother's elevated cortisol levels.[172]

Let me give you some very practical examples of how Christ's Resurrection power is changing me—how my epigenetics are being changed! The first example comes from my physical condition. My battle with Parkinson's has brought about some amazing transformations in my life. I had never realized that I had harbored a deep prejudice toward disabled people. All biases originate from fear and I came to realize

---

[169] Randy Jirtle, "The science of hope: an interview with Randy Jirtle," *Epigenomics* (2022) 14(6), 299–302.

[170] Nessa Carey, *The Epigenetics Revolution*, 55.

[171] Endocrine Society. "Babies Show Ripple Effects Of Mothers Stress From 9/11 Trauma." *ScienceDaily*. www.sciencedaily.com/releases/2005/05/050503153904.htm.

[172] Matas-Blanco, Cristina, and Rafael A. Caparros-Gonzalez. 2020. "Influence of Maternal Stress during Pregnancy on Child's Neurodevelopment" *Psych* 2, no. 4: 186-197. https://doi.org/10.3390/psych2040016.

this fact as I found myself attending a boxing class: a boxing class for folks who are battling Parkinson's! While we were standing, about half the class was fighting the uncontrollable symptoms of their hands shaking all the time and the other half had drool running down the side of their mouth.

Nowadays, I find myself filled with compassion as I look at my teammates. Some of them have become my heroes. "Fast Eddy" shows up every day, even though he can only take tiny steps when he tries to move forward; and I have to help him find the next exercise station because the disease has affected his mental abilities as well. I call him Fast Eddy because Parkinson's causes people to freeze; at times, I literally can't take a step forward. This is incredibly frustrating because I used to be a college gymnast yet, at times, I will be stuck outside an elevator unable to step forward. With each passing elevator full of folks who find my lack of movement puzzling or humorous, my humility factor deepens. It has grown exponentially in the last year, especially in public.

A second example of Christ's Resurrection power getting worked out in my life came from a moment God spoke to me from His Word and then applied it to me during a Pure Desire group I was leading.

In my devotions one morning, I read the puzzling passage in the first chapter of Job.

> *Then the Lord asked Satan, "Have you noticed my servant, Job? He is the finest man in all the earth. He is blameless—a man of complete integrity. He fears God and stays away from evil."*
>
> *Satan replied to the Lord, "Yes, but Job has good reason to fear God. You have always put a wall of protection around him and his home and his property. You have made him prosper in everything he does. Look how rich he is! But reach out and take away everything he has, and he will surely curse you to your face!"*
>
> *"All right, you may test him," the Lord said to Satan. "Do whatever you want with everything he possesses, but don't harm him physically." So Satan left the Lord's presence.*
>
> JOB 1:8-12 (NLT)

Suddenly, I had one of those Homer Simpson moments! I had never noticed it before; Satan brought an accusation against Job, not based on his actions but on the attitude of his heart. And God rendered a verdict. Job would struggle with sickness and disease. Now let me underline the fact that the illness and disease did not come from the Lord but was the result of a legal case Satan brought against him before God. I began to understand the true nature of the battle that was taking place. I realized individuals could not receive the healing Christ purchased for them on the Cross and released to them through the Resurrection because there can be a case against them in the spiritual realm! This case against us can give the enemy room to continually trip us up.

Then the Holy Spirit reminded me of the compelling and practical insights James gave us into the struggles of Job.

> *"Since each of you are part of God's family, never complain or grumble about each other so that judgment will not come on you, for the true Judge is near and very ready to appear! My brothers and sisters, take the prophets as your mentors. They have prophesied in the name of the Lord, and it brought them great sufferings, yet they patiently endured. We honor them as our heroes because they remained faithful even while enduring great suffering. And you have heard of all that Job went through, and we can now see that the Lord ultimately treated him with wonderful kindness, revealing how tenderhearted he really is!"*
>
> JAMES 5:9-11 (TPT)

James emphasizes how God's ultimate verdict in our lives, like with Job, will be when we receive compassion and grace from the Lord. We can, however, have issues in our lives which give hell grounds to accuse us; even though God has tried to get our attention to our vulnerability.

Once I realized hell was my accuser in the courtrooms of heaven, I was shocked awake! I now knew I had a prejudiced attitude in other areas of my life. In the middle of our weekly check-in in my Pure Desire group, I found myself irritated by one guy's repeated comments about his struggles with fantasy. I was thinking to myself, *Come on, dude, grow up!* This is when I heard the Holy Spirit speak to me in an audible voice, "Why are you so judgmental, Ted? You do the same thing!" Then I almost responded by yelling, "I DO NOT!" I don't know why I reacted this way, other than I was afraid God had spoken so loudly that the group heard it as well. This is when the Holy Spirit moved from preaching to meddling: "Why are you secretly looking forward to picking the mail on your way home after boxing?" BUSTED!

The tenderness of God had broken through in my life. At the same time hell was presenting its case against me before God, it was quietly pumping lies into my well-developed excuse machine. It was dumping Novocaine into my soul as Satan prepared to gut me!

What I was looking forward to seeing in the mail were the ads for male enhancement products. When you turn a certain age, your mailbox is awash with graphic pictures of the incredible stud you can become if you buy their product, including tantalizing illustrations of what could happen to your love life! I had excused reading the ads as just a part of life "as you get older." And, I told this to myself—another shot of Novocaine to my soul. I wasn't looking at porn or masturbating like most guys. And besides, we all will struggle with fantasy in this culture until the day we die!

The words from James 5, "...**the true Judge is near and very ready to appear**," shocked me awake. It became crystal clear to me how Satan is the ultimate sleazeball attorney. The whole time he's telling you everything is fine, he is using the legal system of heaven against you.

I will remember this moment for the rest of my life. When I realized what hell was doing against me, I cried out to God and fantasy lost its grip on my soul at that very moment! I realized the quiet hypocrite I had become. Hell had set the groundwork for my eventual destruction down the road. If I continued swallowing the lies hell was feeding me, it would only be a matter of time and I would see over 40 years of ministry destroyed. I cannot imagine the devastation this would release in the hearts of the men I have mentored. I saw the tenderness of God, my Father! How His goodness had destroyed and exposed the enemy's lies. Many leaders and pioneers I have walked with in the area of sexual addiction recovery have fallen along the way. I now realized how incredibly twisted and stealthy hell is and how I desperately needed to lean into the goodness and tenderness of Jesus. All of this was birthed in a lie: "I can't be free from this; it is something I will just have to live with." **I was stuck and didn't even realize it**!

When I started writing this book over four years ago, I didn't plan on including this part of my story. I just remember writing in the outline the statement, The Resurrection, Chapter 15. During these four years, I have developed a growing frustration over how stuck guys were in the healing process. I mean, why are there so many who aren't getting healed? I had a sense in my Spirit that God would reveal His ultimate answer in this chapter. AND HE DID!

So, where are you stuck in your healing process? It may be evident through a frequent relapse. Or you may be believing hell's lies: "This is something you will just have to live with!" Are you finally to the place where you are not acting out, like I was, but your mind is not free from fantasy?

List the specific area where you are stuck (e.g., in my fantasy life; in my tendency to not be totally honest with my wife.)

01. _____
02. _____
03. _____
04. _____
05. _____

Also list the specific excuses you are making for activities or thoughts which are counter to what God has clearly warned you about. (Such as me looking at male enhancement ads.)

List these excuses even if you now realize hell was using these attitudes or actions to present its case against you. (e.g., I don't do it all the time; it's not that bad. Guys in my group do much worse things than watching porn.)

01. _____

02. _____

03. _____

04. _____

05. _____

A third and final example of how Christ's Resurrection power is at work in my life came shortly after this. Even after all of this, the Holy Spirit wasn't through shocking me; He asked me to read James 5:9-11 again. This time, I read it slowly and out loud. It suddenly hit me what preceded James' comment about the Lord appearing as a judge:

> *Since each of you are part of God's family, never complain or grumble about each other so that judgment will not come on you.*
> **JAMES 5:9 (TPT)**

I hadn't thought about this in over a year, but I had grumbled and complained about a staff member. I had written an email that could function as an igniter for setting ablaze almost anything. I mean, I poured out my anger and frustration!

Once again, I had given Satan and his legal team the data to build an iron-clad case against me. Here is the double bind in all of this: the Lord will allow Satan to bring destruction in our lives when he has a solid case against us. The Lord never desires this to occur, but until the truth of the Cross is enforced in our daily lives, the enemy wins the case.

The moment Jesus cried out from the Cross, "It is finished,"[173] He declared every legal requirement was met for reconciling and reclaiming all things back to God. But the challenge of the Cross is for us to enforce the fact of Christ's sacrifice. The verdict that we are no longer under a curse is settled in heaven, but until it is implemented, it has no power. Why do we see a jarring discrepancy between what we say we believe and what we experience? Because we haven't applied the power of Christ to our specific situation and allowed Him to transform us into a new man.

For me, this meant a realization that I needed to immediately apologize to the person I had attacked through my email. I didn't want to allow hell to win a single case against me.

---

[173] John 19:30.

This is the stunning truth about the Resurrection—though the ultimate and final battle has been won by Christ, the effects of that victory may not be realized in our life if we are still giving Satan places to accuse us.

So considering all this, what do you need to do to deal with these places in your life, as God has been doing in my life? Is there anyone to whom you need to write a letter of apology? What steps do you need to take to deal with an area where Satan could build a case against you? What are the unredeemed corners of your life? List them below, along with the steps you will take and the dates for completing these steps.

I need to:

Steps I need to take:

Date for completing these steps:

I need to:

___

Steps I need to take:

___

Date for completing these steps:

___

I need to:

_____
_____
_____
_____
_____
_____
_____
_____

Steps I need to take:

_____
_____
_____
_____
_____
_____
_____
_____
_____
_____

Date for completing these steps:

_____

In the next chapter, we will discover an even more stunning truth about the Resurrection!

BE PREPARED TO SHARE WITH YOUR GROUP YOUR ANSWERS TO THE QUESTIONS IN THIS CHAPTER.

CHAPTER 16
THE STUNNING TRUTH ABOUT THE RESURRECTION—PART 2

You and I can be trapped on the merry-go-round of relapse for years—whether that relapse is our old addiction, anger, or another form of escape and numbing out. In order to step off the merry-go-round, we must break the generational curse and eliminate the case the enemy has against us.

> *We acknowledge our wickedness, O Lord, and the iniquity of our fathers, for we have sinned against you.*
>
> JEREMIAH 14:20 (ESV)

This verse graphically illustrates how the evil of our fathers can cause a perversion of our desires and longings. Thus, we are being pulled by temptation based on what our fathers and mothers allowed in their lives. It also gives hell the legal right to attack us. Once I understood this marvelous truth, I finally realized why sexual health had been such a battle for me through the years.

So how do we experience the freedom Christ purchased for us on the Cross? Revelation 12 speaks powerful about Christ's victory over our accuser:

> *It has come at last—salvation and power and the Kingdom of our God and the authority of his Christ. For the accuser of our brothers and sisters has been thrown down to earth—the one who accuses them before our God day and night. And they have defeated him by the blood of the Lamb and by their testimony.*
>
> REVELATION 12:10-11 (NLT)

In my thinking, I had put this passage exclusively within the context of Christ's final coming. But once I understood the meaning of the phrase "the one who accuses," I realized how far off I was in comprehending the passage. The phrase refers to someone who accuses you in a court of law.[174] I wondered, *Why would the writer use an Old Testament legal term in Revelations 12, which is about the final defeat of Satan?*

Then it dawned on me; I was thinking as if I was ignorant of what Christ had purchased for me on the Cross. Hell was defeated at the Cross. Satan was thrown out of heaven over two thousand years ago. Jesus Christ and the Holy Spirit are now our intercessors forever replacing the accuser in the courtroom of heaven! Hell is trying to bring accusations against us through our bloodline (family of origin). But Hebrews proclaims that the blood Jesus sprinkled for us in heaven **is still speaking for us today**!

> *And we have come to Jesus who established a new covenant with his blood sprinkled upon the mercy seat; blood that continues to speak from heaven, "forgiveness," a better message than Abel's blood that cries from the earth, "justice."*
> HEBREWS 12:24 (TPT)

So, how do we experience the freedom Christ purchased for us? How do we break the endless cycle of relapse? The next verse in Revelation 12 gives us a clear path to freedom.

> *They triumphed over him by the blood of the Lamb and by the word of their testimony; they did not love their lives so much as to shrink from death."*
> REVELATION 12:11 (NIV)

Revelations 12:11 identifies the three things that will enable us to win every case hell would bring against us in courts of heaven.

#1. The Blood of the Lamb

Christ's work on the Cross was the most significant legal transaction of all time. It would grant God the Father the legal right to forgive and cleanse all our sins, forever. It became the basis for the restoration of all people, and even creation would be redeemed.[175] We can never underestimate the power of the blood of the Lamb on the Cross.

---

[174] Colin Brown, *Dictionary of New Testament Theology: Volume 1* (Grand Rapids: Zondervan Publishing House, 1986), 83-84.

[175] Romans 8:21-24.

#2. The Word of their Testimony

The Passion Translation says: "They conquered him completely through the blood of the Lamb and the powerful word of his testimony."

The Passion Translation changes "the word of their testimony" to simply "of his testimony." Why the change? The simple fact is that we will never be strong enough to conquer the devil (our testimony) entirely on our own. This is why one of the hardest things to do in life is to be saved by grace! Christ's testimony and His grace in our lives IS our testimony—PERIOD!

#3. Not Shrink from Death

This is an amazing truth to grasp. When we understand the power of God's grace in our lives, it gives us the courage to stand boldly and face our fears and problems rather than running from them. In the past, our addiction was a way to escape pain and metaphorical death. But as we experience the Resurrection, we emerge changed.

This was illustrated recently as I talked with a young husband who had relapsed again. I started with my standard questions, "Have you done a crash site investigation?" To which he replied, "I knew you would ask that question. So I completed one."

I questioned him further: "So what did you discover? How did the enemy set you up?" He then started laying out a long list of things that had hit him during the day. His wife had recently been very irritable. He added, with their son in the ICU, he could understand why she might be on edge. He finished his comments with, "I went online looking for a banner for our son's welcome home party. But in the process, I ended up watching porn, and once I went that far, I just kept on going and binging on porn."

I asked, "You stated your wife was edgy. Did she say anything to you that triggered you?"

"Yes, her words hurt me deeply," he responded with tears in his eyes. "She made a comment which seemed to demean all of my efforts to help her!"

Then I asked him the critical question: "Let's rewind the tape; what could you have done that would have prevented you from diving into the old relapse cycle?" He shrugged his shoulders and gave me the typical "I don't know" look. He still couldn't explain why he had binged on porn. I reminded him of the vows he made in his life. He was afraid he would never be good enough and he viewed asking for help as an expression of weakness.

I went on to explain: "When you are under pressure, the smartest thing you can do is choose to act in a manner that is opposed to those two curses you have spoken over yourself for years. If you could rewind the incident a bit, a better approach might be for you to be vulnerable with your wife, choosing to be honest and expressing how her words hurt you. Secondly, you could have shared with her how stressed you were when you found out today that your job may be in jeopardy and you were afraid of what that might mean financially for the family. You didn't say a word about the fears you were battling, but if you had, you would have experienced a radically different outcome. Diane and I have discovered that we can face anything together. If we let hell tear us apart because we are not leaning on each other, we will end up arguing over absolutely everything."

I continued to speak truth into his life: "You allowed her words to hurt you and didn't say anything to her, then you closed yourself off and began to feel that you were ENTITLED. **Your fears were controlling you.** When you are angry, you can end up totally out of touch and ignorant of the fact that your fears are driving you. As a result, you will act out and be unable to tell me why you violated all your boundaries."

This young man was able to see that Christ's healing work meant he could face these fears, and vulnerabilities, and not shrink back from them. Rather than protecting his life and reputation, he could lose his life in protecting others.

"Fear not..." This command appears frequently in Scripture. When we find ourselves staring at fear and trying to hide the fact that we are afraid, this is when our loving Father points us to the splattered blood on the splintered beams and gently says to us, "Don't be afraid. Don't shrink back from death. My blood and my testimony is with you!"

When do you get angry to cover your fears?

_____
_____
_____
_____
_____
_____

How is Father God challenging you to become vulnerable in your life instead of puffing up or shrinking back?

_____
_____
_____
_____
_____
_____

> Where do you need to apply Christ's challenge "Do not fear" in your family relationships?

_____
_____
_____
_____

Abraham Lincoln's response to a Union soldier who was arrested for desertion in the Civil War comes to mind. The soldier was sentenced to death, but when his appeal for clemency found its way to the President's desk, he granted him a pardon.[176] The young man returned to his unit and served faithfully for the rest of the war. He died in the last battle. The signed letter of the President was discovered in his breast pocket. Close to the heart of the young warrior were his commander-in-chief's words of pardon. He had found the courage to face his fears. He had found the courage of grace.

In Luke 23, the Roman centurion who supervised the execution of Christ had never heard Him speak. He never saw any of His miracles. He only witnessed the way He died. A man's real character is revealed as he faces pain and betrayal. And Christ's nature was so powerfully impacting on this jaded old combat vet that he cried out, "Surely this was a righteous man."[177]

What we see here is how **absolute power reveals absolutely**. There was only one who had absolute power and it's God. If you look at the life of Christ, you see the stunning truth: He came to the place of having absolute power, yet **it did not corrupt Him**.[178] In the life of Christ, we see that having authority doesn't change you. Instead, it reveals the real you.

Have you ever known someone who received a little power and they changed? And they changed even more when they received more power? And you found yourself thinking, *I don't know who they are anymore!* The truth is, for the first time, you finally understand who they really are. What do I mean? Let's look at this exquisite moment in the life of Christ.

> *It was just before the Passover Festival. Jesus knew that the hour had come for him to leave this world and go to the Father. Having loved his own who were in the world, he loved them to the end. The evening meal was in progress, and the devil had already prompted Judas, the son of Simon Iscariot, to betray Jesus.*

---

[176] A. Gordon Nasby, *1041 Sermon Illustrations, Ideas, and Expositions: Treasury of the Christian World* (Grand Rapids: Baker Books, 1976), 244.

[177] Luke 23:47 (NIV).

[178] Contrary to the phrase "...absolute power corrupts absolutely" made by historian Lord Action (1834-1902) in a letter to Bishop Mandell Creighton regarding the abuse of power.

***Jesus knew that the Father had put all things under his power**, and that he had come from God and was returning to God; so he got up from the meal, took off his outer clothing, and wrapped a towel around his waist. After that, he poured water into a basin and began to wash his disciples' feet, drying them with the towel that was wrapped around him.*

JOHN 13:1-5 (NIV)

Jesus now had all power; and he understood who he was and where he was going. The Hero's Journey is now clearly before him. Let me ask you a question: what would you do if you knew you had all the power? What would be your first act if you had unlimited power? Give yourself a huge mansion and a big boat? Appoint yourself president and fix the world's problems? Destroy terrorism and wars?

What did Jesus do with absolute power? He gets up and washes the disciples' feet! When Jesus had absolute power, what is the first thing he does? He serves us. This, my friends, is truly The Way of the Warrior.

We can understand and worship Christ as the One who claimed to be before time and was higher than death—the soaring eagle of eternity! That is usually not a hard concept to accept. **But the thing that messes with our minds is the truth that God is more humble than us!** He allowed a minimum-wage Roman soldier to drive nails into his wrists. He associated freely with notorious sinners and the sexually broken. His humility models true heroism.

Recently, I realized that after Jesus received all power, he didn't perform a single miracle. Why receive all power then stop doing miracles? You see, He saved the best for last. Oh yes, I am referring to the Resurrection. That was impressive, but it wasn't the most striking thing. The greatest miracle performed was the one that didn't just defy the laws of nature but challenged everything we would have expected. Jesus allowed Himself to be killed, the God who is life experienced Death, so that through His sacrifice, we might live! **This is the miracle of Jesus' absolute power—He served us, which is the stunning truth of the Resurrection!**

The Mighty Warrior Finds Honor in Service

God, who is all-powerful, will never demand that you love Him. God, who is all-powerful, will always give you the freedom to choose. **God is not motivated by His power; He is only motivated by His love.** He only uses His power to respond to your cry for help.

When you are tired of drowning in your shame and guilt, He freely forgives you. When you are finally done with the crazy relapse cycle and you sincerely reach out to Him, He brings His power to change the course of your life and destiny. When you are exhausted from fighting the war within yourself, by yourself, His power brings support and rest for your weary soul. When you are frustrated in your battle with anger that seems to suddenly erupt, tearing apart the people you love, He comes without judgment to bring His peace to you. **God will only use His power to set you free, make you whole, and restore your humanity. He will never force His rule upon you. Instead, He will fight for you and not against you.**

How would you like to respond to this incomprehensible love? His love has set you free from the wounds that gave birth to the crippling vows which kept you stuck in life! His love sets you free from the corrosive grip of anger. His love has given you wings to soar far above the fears that once kept you grounded.

In the space below, take some time to express your thanks to Christ in a prayer.

MY PRAYER OF THANKS[179]

_____
_____
_____
_____
_____
_____
_____
_____
_____
_____
_____
_____
_____
_____
_____
_____
_____

[179] In Appendix A, I have included sample prayers that deal with breaking vows and generational curses. And these prayers would also serve as a template to develop prayers to confront Satan and any charges he would bring against you in the courtroom of heaven.

If Christ used His power in this way, He truly shows us The Way of the Warrior. What this ultimately means for you and me is that when we experience His Resurrection power in our life, it is so that we can serve others. We are resurrected for a higher purpose—the purpose of loving others like Christ loved us!

How does this happen? For the rest of this chapter, let's look at three powerful ways you serve others through the deep, internal work you are doing.

Developing Empathy

In the previous chapter, I asked a challenging question: Is there anyone to whom you need to write a letter of apology?

In counseling, Diane and I lead couples through the disclosure process, which includes the betrayed partner writing an Emotional Impact Letter, and then the addict spouse writing an Emotional Restitution Letter in response to their partner.

In taking couples through this process, there are two foundational steps an addicted husband must experience, especially if he is caught in an endless cycle of relapse. The key here is understanding that sexual addiction is a family system problem. This means the addictive insanity has deeply impacted the marriage relationship. Once you realize this statement is true, then it makes sense why the man needs to write a heartfelt, vulnerable, and emotionally connected letter of apology to his wife. In other words, he starts to develop real empathy. Then the marriage can usually turn around; it doesn't matter how deep the wounds from the past may be.

I mentioned there are two critical steps that must occur, and the first step is the tough one! Because denial is so strong, we ask the husband to read his wife's Emotional Impact Letter ***every day***. We are praying God will do what only He can do, which is the second step. That God would lovingly break his heart and give him the supernatural gift of empathy. **Empathy is not just feeling sorry for the pain the addiction has inflicted on his wife.** It is something far more powerful and beautiful. **It is the gift of understanding how she feels!**

Whether you have received an Emotional Impact Letter or not, you must come to grips with how deeply your behavior has impacted your partner and continually work on having empathy for her. Through betrayal, a partner loses her sense of trust and safety, and possibly her youth, the loss of finances, and more. This may also include feelings of isolation she has suffered and how crippled she felt because she couldn't share with anyone what her husband was doing; especially if he was a pastor or involved in a Christian ministry.

You may or may not be a pastor or involved in Christian ministry, but when have you felt terrified or worried about someone finding out about your addiction? What have you done to cover your tracks? Have you ever deflected blame on your wife to make her the problem?

_____
_____
_____
_____

Share an incident where you tried to hide your addictive behavior by minimizing, denying, or blaming your wife.

_____
_____
_____
_____

How are you doing at having empathy toward your wife? How would you rate yourself?

_____
_____
_____
_____

Understand the Impact of Trauma on the Brain

One of the most powerful ways we can develop greater empathy for our partner is to understand how our betrayal has had a physical impact on her brain. I will often ask men, "How many of you found it helpful to discover that you were dealing with a brain problem in your struggle to get free? It is not just about trying harder." Most of the guys raise their hands or nod their heads in agreement.

Gentlemen, what we need to do now is take our comprehension of the human brain much deeper. Let's talk about what happens to your wife's brain when she discovers the truth about what you were doing when you were in your addiction. As we'll discuss, recent research has revealed why your wife wrestles so intensely with letting go of your past behavior and forgiving you. When your wife discovered what you were doing when you told her you had to work late, it devastated her to realize you were watching porn at the job site. Or you were visiting a massage parlor or having an ongoing affair with a coworker or whatever you were doing instead of being faithful to her. She was thrown into deep trauma!

Trauma affects the female brain in three powerful ways. **First of all, it triggers the amygdala.**[180] This area of the brain determines if she feels safe. The question she will immediately ask herself when you are working late: *Is our relationship safe or is he lying to me and acting out? Can I trust his promises?* When she discovers you were lying to her for _____ years (you fill in the blank), the amygdala becomes fear central! The result is the limbic part of her brain starts sending alarm signals throughout her entire brain and her higher-level thinking parts shut down. She will lose the ability to reason. Have you noticed how hard it is to reason with your wife when she feels triggered?

At this point, all the men are frantically nodding their heads in agreement.

The second area is her insula.[181] This is the area of the brain involved in interoception, which is one's ability to feel into internal experiences and connect them with internal sensations. For example, when you feel hungry, warm, or jittery, these are typical examples of interoception. Trauma dysregulates this part of her brain, making it very difficult for her to identify and manage her emotions. For instance, she can suddenly become furious at you and she may not even know why.[182]

Now every man is listening and fully engaged!

The third piece in the trauma puzzle is what has taken place in her hippocampus which is her memory center, as well as the timekeeper.[183] This part of her brain takes short-term memory and moves it into long term memory, which provides her with a sense of history. This part of the mind has been so affected by trauma it may even shrink, resulting in an innocent situation perceived or seen as being dangerous. This is why a combat veteran can hit the ground at the sound of a car backfiring. I once jumped into a large metal garbage container at the sound of a siren from the local fire station in Wilmore, Kentucky, and this was three years after returning from Vietnam![184] The reason for such illogical responses is that the amygdala's warning

---

[180] Protopopescu, X., Pan,H., Tuescher, Cloitre, M. (2005). *Differential time courses and specificity of amygdala activity in post-traumatic stress disorder subjects and normal control subjects.* Biological Psychiatry, *57(5), 464-473.*

[181] Jennifer Sweeton, *Trauma Treatment Toolbox: 165 Brain-Changing Tips, Tools & Handouts to Move Therapy Forward* (Eau Claire: PESI Publishing, 2019), 3-36.

[182] Simpson, A., Strigo, I.A., Matthews, S.C., Paulus, M. (2009). Initial evidence of a failure to activate right anterior Insula during affective set-shifting in PTSD. *Psychosomatic Medicine*, 71(4) 373.

[183] Jennifer Sweeton, *Trauma Treatment Toolbox*, 9-10.

[184] Ted Roberts, *Pure Desire: How One Man's Triumph Can Help Others Break Free From Sexual Temptation* (Raleigh: Regal House Publishing, 1999), 200.

signals reverberate through the brain. They are overpowering the prefrontal cortex to such an extent that all you do is REACT! **If something doesn't make sense in your life, it is usually limbic in origin.**

So, gentlemen, do you want me to translate all of this neurochemistry into something that will help you better understand your wife? Consider this: it would be as if you walked up to the large file cabinet, which is filled with your wife's memories or her history, and threw a grenade into it! The trauma she experienced once she found out about your secret sexual behaviors blew her memories apart! This is why she can become so insecure. She can't trust her perception because she thought everything was fine, but then found out you were lying to her! How could she have been so naive? She has also lost a sense of herself. We understand who we are through the historical sequence of events constructed in our minds. So now, who is she? She thought you loved her; but those events which used to build her view of herself, have proved to be false.

One wife powerfully expressed it, "As I look at our family pictures now, I realize it was all a lie. I thought he loved me, but he was more interested in spending time with _____." (You can put the name of your addictive behavior in the blank, your favorite porn site, the name of the coworker you were having an affair with, or the name of the massage parlor.)

I don't bring up the reality of your wife's experience to condemn you or trigger shame within you. Instead, to highlight the difficult task she faces in learning to trust you again. Therefore, two things are real:

- If discovery or full disclosure has taken place recently, she is probably going to wrestle severely over the next 12 months to forgive and trust you.
- You will have to **earn her trust**! Therefore, when you react in anger toward her lack of trust in you, guess what? The relationship goes back to **square one**.

> How will this new information concerning the impact of betrayal on your wife help you deal with the tough times you may have together?

___

> How have you been irritated with your wife when she brings up your past betrayal?

___

Describe a recent incident where you were irritated with her for bringing it up.

_____
_____
_____
_____

How have you been upset with her when she becomes emotional and you feel as if you can't reason with her?

_____
_____
_____
_____
_____

Have you grown in having empathy for your wife? Circle the response/score that best answers this question.

not much	slightly	okay	better	much better
1	2	3	4	5

Ask your wife how she would score you.

_____
_____

What could you do to respond better the next time these situations occur?

_____
_____
_____
_____

Breaking Inner Vows

There is one other issue I believe can set us free to serve others like Christ, the ultimate Hero. This issue also lies at the core of why some guys never seem to get out of relapse. I can share all the information I just shared with you about how the guy's actions have affected his wife and it still doesn't seem to help. It is as if they are stuck spiritually! With regard to my own anger, I came to realize nothing seemed to help, no matter how hard I tried to change. It didn't matter how many times I declared my total commitment not to lash out in anger at those I loved. I would find myself relapsing in anger and once again trying to dig myself out of that familiar pit of shame. And the crazy thing about my relapses was I loved Jesus more than I ever had! I was missing something in the spiritual realm.

As I began to desperately pray for the Holy Spirit to open my eyes, I just happened to run across the following comment in *The Genesis Process*, "Inner vows can become mandates, which act like self curses...[they] become subconscious and do not go away with time, **but are like a contract and must be renounced and broken**."[185] I must have read this statement a hundred times before as we had led couples through the healing process. But this time, words came alive to me; it was as if they jumped off the page and grabbed hold of my mind! I realized why I had struggled with anger in my heart for such a long time.

Trauma had burned a moment from my past into my limbic brain. In the middle of the night, I was jolted awake by the screams of my mother. My sixth stepfather (out of seven) had gotten bored with just beating her. He decided to add a little more drama to the evening by dragging Mom into the bathroom to drown her. I exploded out of my bed to save her. A vicious backhand from my stepfather abruptly truncated my rescue efforts. He knocked me down the hallway, and as I staggered to my feet, a brutal punch impacted my face. I laid sprawled across my bedroom floor. I tried to stagger to my feet, while blood poured from my mouth. He towered over me, pointed his finger at me, and bellowed, "If you get up, I will kill you!"

I am not stupid; I stayed down! But inside me, I made a vow that set the course for my life for the next 30 years. I promised myself: *I will never let another man treat me like that EVER AGAIN!* This was when I finally realized the source of my deep abiding anger. Sports in high school and college were not just about playing a game. It was about beating other men. Volunteering for a combat assignment was not just about serving my country; it was ultimately about proving I was a man! The anger that exploded in my heart that one traumatic and dark night, set the course of my life for the next 30 years.

When we recognize and renounce these vows, we can find a new freedom to serve others. Our purpose in life can shift entirely! Rather than beating other men, the Lord has made it my mission to love them and help them find freedom from addiction. What mission could God unleash in your life?

---

[185] Michael Dye, *The Genesis Process: For Change Groups, Book 1 and 2, Individual Workbook* (Auburn: Double Eagle Industries, 2012), 127.

What vows have you made out of the pain of your past? (e.g., I will never trust a woman; if I am vulnerable, I will get hurt; my worth is about my performance; asking for help is a sign of weakness; whatever I do, it will not be good enough.)

01. _____

02. _____

03. _____

What happened in your life that caused you to make these vows?

_____
_____
_____

How have the vows you made affected your marriage and family?

_____
_____
_____

Renounce these inner vows in a prayer and ask Christ to fill you with a new power to live in freedom from their impact.

_____
_____
_____
_____

Based on what you've learned so far, how is it helping you become a Compassionate Warrior? Be specific in your answer.

_____
_____
_____

BE PREPARED TO SHARE WITH YOUR GROUP YOUR ANSWERS TO THE QUESTIONS IN THIS CHAPTER.

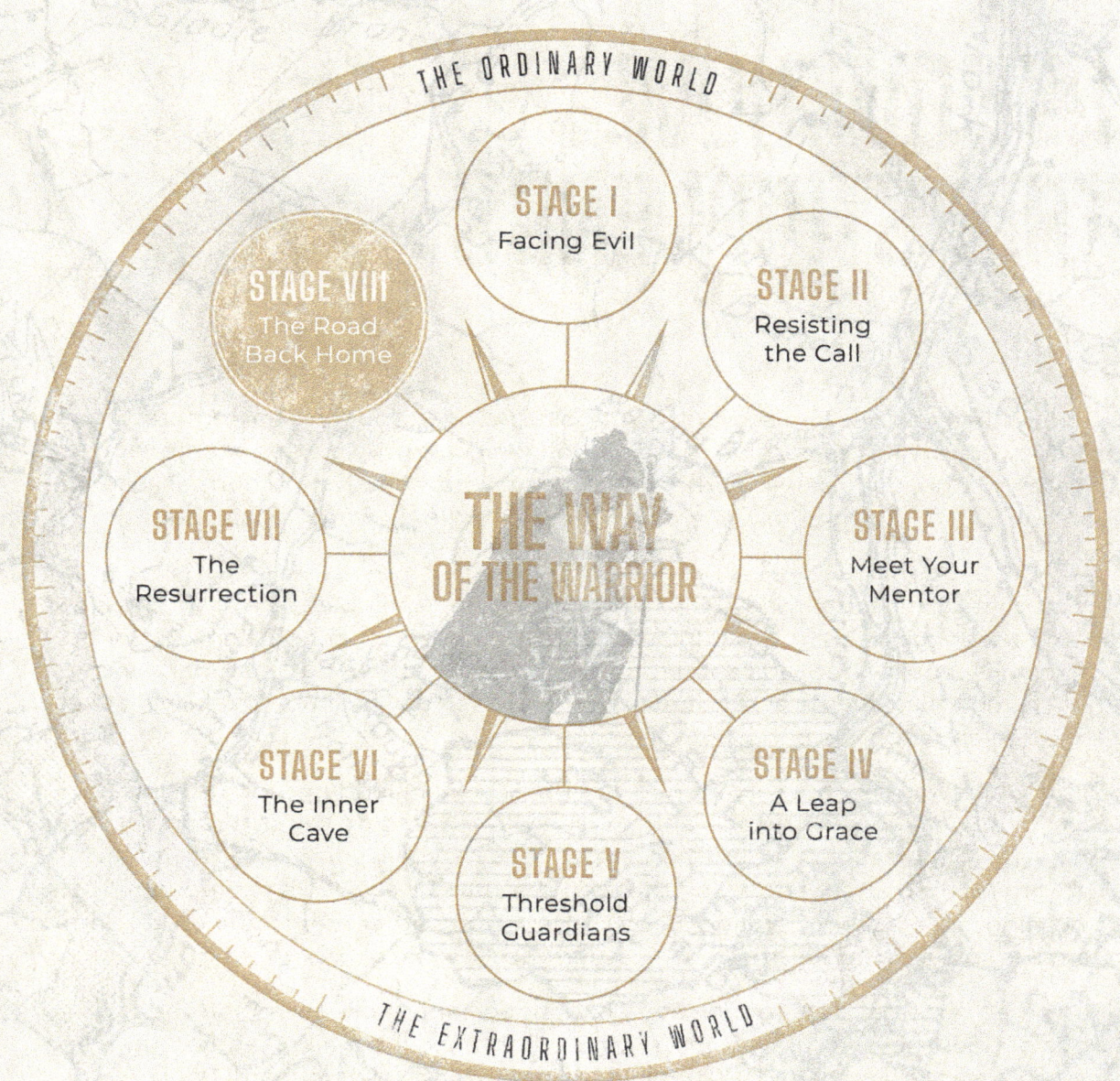

STAGE VIII

THE ROAD BACK HOME

CHAPTER 17
I KNOW HOW THIS STORY ENDS

There is no faster way to discover the purpose of God in your life than embracing the daily opportunities to serve those around you. When we do this—center our life around Christ and serving others—we create a new and lasting normal as a transformed, renewed hero. We are living in the "ordinary world" again, but as a forever changed man! This is The Road Back Home.

Unfortunately, for some men, the shame surrounding their past sexual sin causes them to see their healing as a personal issue. It is never just about them. But often, they don't want to openly talk about how God brought them out of sexual bondage; there is too much shame associated with their past. They hesitate to take, what I call, "sweet revenge" on the enemy of their soul.

This is when you take the very point of your past sexual bondage and use it as a devastating weapon against the enemy. One way you can do this is through serving as a leader or coleader of a Pure Desire group. Or maybe leading a *Sexual Integrity 101*[186] group, then afterward taking the men through *Seven Pillars of Freedom*. There is nothing as personally fulfilling in my life as helping other men come to freedom from the sexual struggles they have battled with for years!

Many men hesitate to share their story of bondage and brokenness and the saving grace of God. They withdraw from helping other men who are presently caught in the same trap they escaped. In other words, they don't pay it forward! Paul beautifully expressed this challenge in Scripture:

> *So never be ashamed to tell others about our Lord. And don't be ashamed of me, either, even though I'm in prison for him. With the strength God gives you, be ready to suffer with me for the sake of the Good News. For God saved us and called us to live a holy life. He did this, not because we deserved it, but because*

---

[186] Pure Desire Ministries, *Sexual Integrity 101: an 8-week Study for Men, Women, & Churches* (Troutdale: Pure Desire Ministries International, 2020).

that was his plan from before the beginning of time—to show us his grace through Christ Jesus.

2 TIMOTHY 1:8-9 (NLT)

There was a great deal of shame if you identified with a "jail bird" like Paul. This is precisely why many of his disciples pulled back. I have seen a lot of men never come to the freedom God has set aside for them because they hide from being identified with those who struggle with sexual sin in their life.

You may be at a place where you're thinking, *Yeah, service to others, I will get there someday.* It is critical to realize this way of thinking is a refusal of the call of God on your life! You are here for a reason. You were created for a purpose. The choice is yours. You can embrace your role and the unique gift from God in your sexual health and bring meaning to yourself and your world, or you can opt out.

You see a classic picture of sacrifice in the movie, *Terminator 2*,[187] where the robot hero (played by Arnold Schwarzenegger) must sacrifice himself to prevent the ultimate villain, Skynet, from eventually ruling the world. And at a deeper level, the teenager, John Connor, must sacrifice part of himself—his mentor/father figure—by allowing the Terminator to leap to his death.

There is a scene in the first *Star Wars*[188] movie where I always find myself shouting out loud for joy when I watch it. Han Solo is being his normal self-centered, deceptive self, as he turns his back on the rebel's desperate attempt to take out the Death Star. He is essentially taking the money and running. In stark contrast, Luke suits up and straps into his awesome looking X-Wing Starfighter to take on the Death Star. The rebels are obviously outnumbered and have little, if any, chance of taking out the armor-plated monster of the Empire. The rebels are fighting courageously but the enemy's defenses are decimating the X-Wing Starfighters. Finally, Luke breaks through and gets a chance to take out the Death Star—his one-in-a-million shot to somehow pull it off.

Things get really tense as Darth Vader closes in on Luke's six o'clock, ready for the kill shot. Then, at the last second, who shows up? Han Solo comes streaking across the night sky, flying the Millennium Falcon with guns blazing to cover Luke! As a result, Darth Vader's TIE Fighter is sent spinning out of control! As Han zooms off, he encourages Luke to take the shot. Han Solo's showing up at the last possible moment graphically illustrates how he has finally changed and is now willing to risk his life for a just cause. He has become a true warrior of the heart.

---

[187] *Terminator2: Judgment Day*, directed by James Cameron (Los Angeles: Carolco Pictures, 1991), film.

[188] *Star Wars: Episode IV - A New Hope*, directed by George Lucas (San Francisco: Lucasfilm, 1977), film.

Where and when did you realize God will never give up on you?

What group of people has God placed on your heart to help in the future?
Where are you going to take "sweet revenge" on the enemy?

What next step could you begin taking NOW in this direction?

My wife, Diane, and I have been married over 54 years and there is one thing she still does that drives me crazy. She loves to tell me the WHOLE STORY. At times, especially when I am tired and it has been a long day, I find myself pleading with her: "Give me the bottom line! Please, I don't need all the details. Just tell me how the story ends!"

However, when it comes to King David, it's precisely the opposite—I can't get enough details! I love his story because he is an incredibly complex human being. For example, his relationship with the Lord is amazing and never ceases to deeply move me. Yet, there are so many flaws deep within him that he also remains a mystery. How can he be so gracious to Mephibosheth on the one hand,[189] and then on the other, order the execution of Bathsheba's husband, Uriah, on the battlefield?[190]

I have lived long enough to realize the most consistent thing about this world has to be its inconsistency! Evil can live paradoxically close to goodness. At times, it seems that only a thin curtain separates the two. Given the right temptation, at the right moment, attacked at the weakest link in our inner brokenness, there is hardly a man alive who wouldn't live out his vilest fantasies. Once these hidden factors line up in our life, we can also become frighteningly inconsistent as well. As a result, one moment in our life can usher in an incredible victory and the next a crushing defeat. It can feel like the introductory lines for the old ABC sports show: **"Spanning the globe to bring you the constant variety of sports, the thrill of victory, and the agony of defeat!"**[191]

But the one thing that continually amazes me is God's positive evaluation of David's life once he had hung up his cleats and finished his Hero's Journey, despite all of his inconsistencies.

> *"David, of course, **having completed the work God set out for him**, has been in the grave, dust, and ashes, a long time now. But the One God raised up— no dust and ashes for him! I want you to know, my very dear friends, that it is on account of this resurrected Jesus that the forgiveness of your sins can be promised. He accomplishes, in those who believe, everything that the Law of Moses could never make good on. But everyone who believes in this raised-up Jesus is declared good and right and whole before God."*
>
> ACTS 13:36-39 (MSG)

The reason I find Father God's evaluation of David's life so amazing is that David had fallen in his life in ways that made my issues look like a minor bump on the road of life. Now put these two truths together. First, how David had a habit of messing up his life big time; and second, despite the incredibly destructive choices he made, by the grace of God, David finished the Hero's Journey very well. He was able to hear his heavenly Father say to him, "Well done faithful servant." I don't know how you feel about the paradox of these two truths colliding against one another, but it gives a mess up like me **tremendous hope**!

Throughout this chapter, the questions we are going to answer are, How did David pull this off? How did he recover from his frequent relapses to finish so well? I think there were **three things he got right** which gave him **phenomenal resilience**. No

---

[189] 2 Samuel 9.

[190] 2 Samuel 11.

[191] *ABC's Wide World of Sports*, Jim McKay (United States, American Broadcasting Company, 1961), TV.

matter how many times David got knocked down or he knocked himself down, he always found the ability to get up one more time! So, the critical question is: how do we learn this same godly resilience that David had?

I've developed a rather unique habit during the summer. I can't even remember how it started, but when it finally stops raining in Oregon, I always begin to read through the Psalms of David. It's hard to describe exactly what takes place in my soul. But as I read through the 73 Psalms ascribed to David, it is as if I am listening to a symphony orchestra of the Holy Spirit and the string section is reflecting every note of praise and prayer. The woodwinds are telling of David's triumphs and troubles. And the percussion and brass are pounding out the deep resonant moments of his gladness and sadness and his hopes and fears. But above all else, I sense **a man who sincerely sees and understands himself from God's viewpoint**.

If I could get a man to see one thing that would increase his chances of walking in freedom, it would be for him to **grasp the power of the promises God has spoken over his life**!

The First Step in Building Resilience

The **first step in building resilience comes from finally seeing and understanding who we are from God's perspective**. It is a challenging task for a guy to make such a severe adjustment in his outlook concerning himself. The hardest part of the transition is learning to be gracious with ourselves.

I still struggle with this. It was not something I naturally did because my inner critic's voice grew so strong through the years. It was something I've had to learn. After all, I had spent years trying to be free from my bondage by working harder.

There is a fantastic example in David's life of the kind of freedom and joy God would bring into our lives as we learn to **dance with him.**

> *Now King David was told, "The Lord has blessed the house of Obed-edom and all that belongs to him, because of the ark of God." So David went and brought up the ark of God from the house of Obed-edom into the City of David with rejoicing and gladness. And when those who were carrying the ark of the Lord [by its poles] had gone six paces, he sacrificed an ox and a fatling. And David was dancing before the Lord with great enthusiasm, and David was wearing a linen ephod [a priest's upper garment]. So David and all the house of Israel were bringing the ark of the Lord up [to the City of David] with shouts [of joy] and with the sound of the trumpet.*
>
> *Then, as the ark of the Lord came into the City of David, Michal, Saul's daughter [David's wife], looked down from the window above and saw King David*

leaping and dancing before the Lord; and she felt contempt for him in her heart [because she thought him undignified].

2 SAMUEL 6:12-16 (AMP)

I can imagine how that parade must have appeared. David had the ark of the covenant loaded on a custom-built cart and it was joined with horns, harps, cymbals, and psalteries. But out front of it all was David, high stepping like the drum major of the Tuskegee University band leading the Crimson Pipers in their victory march. With trumpets blaring and the drums and cymbals pounding in concussive rhythm the royal redhead was lost in the celebration of the moment.[192] The amazing thing was how the two of them cut loose! God and David were whirling around together in such a passion, they caught fire and it resulted in such an intense flame that would light the way for one who would be known as the Son of David. Jesus, who was the Messiah came a thousand years later!

For years, I have desired to be so in love with Father God, like David, but it was blocked for me until I realized I had made a classic mistake. Like walking in sexual health, I thought it was up to me. I thought it was all about me trying harder. David grasped that it was never about trying harder. What he understood about God's grace enabled him to withstand even the contempt filled comments and looks from his wife.

This Psalm of David helps us understand how David saw himself before God:

I have called upon You, for You will answer me, God;
Incline Your ear to me, hear my speech.
Show Your wonderful faithfulness,
Savior of those who take refuge at Your right hand
From those who rise up against them.
Keep me as the apple of the eye;
Hide me in the shadow of Your wings

PSALM 17:6-8 (NASB)

David describes himself as the "apple" of God's eye. This was a poetic way—even thousands of years ago—of describing someone as being very close, and valued, by another person. David understood God's love for him so deeply that he danced in His presence despite the contempt of others. When we live in the truth of God's love for us, we can have the same kind of resilience that David developed.

---

[192] The term used to describe David is abmon^i meaning "ruddy," implying that David had a red complexion or hair. Now I seriously doubt it is describing an Irish redhead like myself, but there must have been a reddish tone to his dark complexion.

The Second Step in Building Resilience

In verses 1-2 of this Psalm, David does an amazing thing that I think kept him sane in such a crazy time:

> *Hear a just cause, O LORD, give heed to my cry;*
> *Give ear to my prayer, which is not from deceitful lips.*
> *Let my judgment come forth from Your presence;*
> *Let your eyes look with equity.*
>
> PSALM 17:1-2 (NASB1995)

David was hunted like a criminal despite his innocence. It is obvious in my mind what you should do when a leader like Saul hurls a spear at your head: you pull it out of the wall and throw it back at him, and make sure you don't miss! David realized, though, if he responded by hurling the spear back at Saul, he would soon end up as crazy as Saul. This is why David's first response to Saul's vicious words and violent spears was to spread the entire matter out before the Lord. He didn't respond by trying to justify himself. Instead, he asked for the Lord's affirmation. In the Lord's presence, we don't have to react in anger defending ourselves or wilting and withdrawing under the pressure of other people's opinions.

This is the **second step in developing godly resilience: believing God will defend us because of how special we are to Him**.

For many, this is almost impossible to do because there is so much unresolved pain over past failure. The open wounds of these unhealed memories from our past can consistently trigger us in the present. This is why self-vindication will never be enough. We need to see ourselves from God's perspective, especially when all hell breaks loose in our lives.

This is why David makes, as we used to say in the fighter pilot community, "a gutsy move." He wanted God to look him in the eye and tell him what he saw. He is opening up himself to the eye of the Lord, which is why he used this unique idiom, *"the apple of your eye."* In Hebrew this means, "the little man of our eye" or "the daughter of the eye."[193]

This metaphor speaks to some of my deepest struggles. If you have ever stood very close to someone and if the light is just right, you will see a reflection of yourself in their eyes. Therefore, when God looks deeply into our lives, He only sees Christ. He is not obsessed with our sins. This is not the focus of His attention. He is essentially saying to each of us, "Quit focusing on your sin, your old self. Christ has already died for all that stuff. I want my Son to become the focus of your attention!"

---

[193] James Johnston, *Preaching the Word: The Psalms Volume 1 - Psalms 1 to 41* (Wheaton: Crossway, 2015), 185.

Now there is also a profound balance point to this truth: God also has never been disillusioned with you either. Do you know why? He has never had any illusions about you. He knows what we are capable of doing and becoming apart from His grace; but only He completely knows us and unconditionally loves us.

> Have you ever struggled, as I did for years, believing God wasn't for you—believing He was against you? When things went wrong in your life, did you suspect God was punishing you for your past mistakes in life? Explain.

> What was your view of God like: an angry dad or a distant uncaring father; or something completely different? What past experience with your earthly father gave you such a negative view of your heavenly Father?

> When was the first time you looked into the face of God and suddenly realized how deeply He loved you?

The delight that God has over each one of us becomes the vaccine for the discouragement that can infect our hearts through the harsh words of those who come against us. We do not see ourselves reflected in God's eyes as the person we have been but, like a miracle, we see the person we can become.

We see this in David's response to King Saul's put down before facing Goliath, *"You are only a boy going up against a seasoned warrior!"*[194] David's response is to agree with Saul's observation concerning his age and the fact that he has never before faced a giant. But he teamed up with the same God when he took out a lion and bear. Therefore, he declares that he knows how this story will end! God had given him a promise that he would be the king one day. He wasn't king yet, but it still sucked for Goliath because David knew how this conflict would end.

> Here is a real challenge in life: when you know how the story will end but you don't have a clue how to get there.

David started as a kind of delivery boy for his dad. Remember, his dad asked him to take some cheese sandwiches down to his brothers on the battlefield? Now if he had been the classic teenager, he would have rolled his eyes and responded with something like, "Oh, come on Dad, you have got to be kidding me!" The result would have been him totally missing the confrontation with Goliath. **If you don't show up and do the ordinary, then God never does the extraordinary in your life.**

Now his brothers had listened to Goliath trash-talk the Israelites for 40 days. So when they heard him once again trash-talk the living God, it sounded normal to them. We can get so used to our dysfunction because we grew up in it and heard it repeated again and again. But David was shocked and asked, "What did that giant say about the living God? And what did King Saul say would be done for the guy who takes out this idiot? Did he say he would get to marry one of his daughters—the hot one? Hey, I know how this story is going to turn out, no one talks about the living God like that!"

And if you read 1 Samuel 17 carefully, you see that there was a delivery boy in the story but it wasn't David—it was Goliath! When you stand facing an enormous problem in the battlefield of life, you need to realize that God is just giving you a preview of how large you are going to become once the battle is over. **Every giant you face in life is a delivery boy from God, holding the answer to the problems you will be facing in the next battle.** David knew how his story would end. This truth will become the core of God's gift of supernatural resilience in your soul!

The Third Step in Building Resilience

As you know, David's life takes some radical turns and twists. In 2 Samuel 19, we find David facing one the most intense reversals in his life. David lost sight of what God told him about how his story would end. He had defeated the enemy, but it turned into shame. He became blind to his victory. In 2 Samuel 19, once again, we see David

---

[194] 1 Samuel 17:33 paraphrase.

saved by a faithful friend who had guts enough to tell him the truth. Joab was the commander of David's army. The scene must have been incredibly gripping; this old battle scarred commander standing boldly before the sobbing king shouting forth commands, "Get up! And get out there!"

You need to thank God for friends who love you enough to tell you what you don't want to hear.

> *Joab went to the house where David was staying and told him: You've made your soldiers ashamed! Not only did they save your life, they saved your sons and daughters and wives as well. You're more loyal to your enemies than to your friends. What you've done today has shown your officers and soldiers that they don't mean a thing to you. You would be happy if Absalom was still alive, even if the rest of us were dead. Now get up! Go out there and thank them for what they did. If you don't, I swear by the Lord that you won't even have one man left on your side tomorrow morning. You may have had a lot of troubles in the past, but this will be the worst thing that has ever happened to you!*
>
> 2 SAMUEL 19:5-7 (CEV)

The critical third step in developing Godly resilience is choosing to boldly confront situations that are opposed to your God-given calling.

Joab's words shocked David into action. He wasn't struggling with just grief; he was dealing with an enormous load of guilt as a dad. Grief and guilt are a toxic mixture. Processing healthy grief will free us to go on living. He was mourning the fact that he hadn't disciplined his children. Especially Absalom, who grew to hate David so deeply he led a rebellion against him and tried to kill him! He was having second thoughts, but it was too late. He saw his sins replicated in his sons' lives. David had allowed some things into his life, little by little, but now it was destroying everything. Once again, David's life becomes a haunting illustration of what *not* to do. His example underlines how it is impossible to sustain our confidence with a flawed character. There is a direct connection between character and confidence.

There is a fascinating sequence of words used by the author to describe David's physical location in chapters 18-19. In 2 Samuel 18:33, we read that the king was shaken and he went up to **the room over the gateway** and wept. In chapter 19, we find Joab coming to that room to confront the king. In verse 8 the author signals an incredible spiritual transition by the change of David's physical location which Joab had triggered through his forceful confrontation.

> *So the king came out and took his place **at the city gate**. Soon everyone knew: "Oh, look! The king has come out to receive us." And his whole army came and presented itself to the king. But the Israelites had fled the field of battle and gone home.*
>
> 2 SAMUEL 19:8 (MSG)

The phrase "the city gate" indicates the place where the business of the city was conducted. In chapter 18, he was located in a room over the city gate. After Joab's terrifying words had shocked David out of his self-pity binge, he took his rightful place. It was his second inauguration. Since David had fled before the return of Absalom—who was crowned as the new king but was killed in the ensuing battle—the people were completely confused as to what they should do. Once David took his seat at the city gate, the army who had melted into the surrounding countryside suddenly returned to celebrate their victory. David got up and took his God-given place, even though he wasn't remotely healed yet. But when he took his seat, all the men came to him. You, like David, may still be hurting; but all the support and weapons you need will show up once you take your seat at the place where God has called you.

David had a defining moment early in life that prepared him for this moment:

God said, "Up on your feet! Anoint him! This is the one."

> *Samuel took his flask of oil and anointed him, with his brothers standing around watching. The Spirit of God entered David like a rush of wind, God vitally empowering him for the rest of his life.*
> 1 SAMUEL 16:12-13 (MSG)

I can only imagine the impact of those words of affirmation and the emotional experience of being anointed as the next king of Israel before his brothers and father, who didn't see anything special about him. Why was David able to get up off the floor after hell took its best shot at him and everyone had discounted him once again? The prophetic experience of Samuel's anointing gave David the power to retake his seat as king despite his failures as a dad.

The thing that makes a personal promise so powerful is the emotional experience of having God encounter us and define who we are from His perspective. When I ask a new client to share his personal promises from God, he will usually give me a short list of Bible verses he likes. I often smile and tell him thanks for the Sunday school verses, but they will be worthless when hell comes knocking at his door. Why is this? For the simple reason, hell's most painful attacks will always be emotional, not intellectual. I will tell the guys to do the assignment again.[195] When they can't share their promises without tears streaming down their face, then I know they are ready to battle hell! In other words, their promises will be worthless if they lack the power of an emotional encounter with the Lord God Almighty.

I am sure David couldn't recall the moment, without tears coming to his eyes, when Samuel poured the anointing oil on his head because God had thundered the words,

---

[195] This assignment is found in the *Seven Pillars of Freedom Workbook*, Pillar 6, Lesson 4.

"This is the one I have chosen!" It had such emotional force because he suffered for years under the brutal rejection of his family of origin. David clearly understood the power of a God-given promise in his life. In Psalms 139:16, he takes this concept to a much deeper level.

> *Your eyes saw my unformed body; all the days ordained for me were written in your book before one of them came to be.*
>
> PSALM 139:16 (NIV)

David is implying that God wrote down in a book in heaven the purpose of each of our lives before we ever existed. He saw not just the number of our days but what we would accomplish in our lives. This is a reflection of what Paul stated in Ephesians 2:10; that we are a result of God's creative efforts. And God prepared the poems of our lives to carry a life-giving impact in our broken world. We find this concept repeatedly in the New Testament.

My passionate prayer is that you will not squander the mercy and grace of God extended to you through His personal promises over you since before the beginning of time. For those who do His will are able to accomplish it because God is at work within us.[196] Sadly, not everyone chooses to live out what was established by God and written down in heaven for their lives. Because of God's great love for us, He allows us to make this choice. In Romans 8:29-30, we find Paul's incredible description of how the intentions of God become realities in our lives.

> *God knew what he was doing from the very beginning. He decided from the outset to shape the lives of those who love him along the same lines as the life of his Son. The Son stands first in the line of humanity he restored. We see the original and intended shape of our lives there in him. After God made that decision of what his children should be like, he followed it up by calling people by name. After he called them by name, he set them on a solid basis with himself. And then, after getting them established, he stayed with them to the end, gloriously completing what he had begun.*
>
> ROMANS 8:29-30 (MSG)

To be honest, I hesitated to quote from The Message translation; but this is such a beautiful rendering of the Greek thought into English. Paul articulates a four-step process of how God's eternal intentions for us are made real in our lives.

---

[196] Philippians 2:13.

GOD KNEW WHAT HE WAS DOING FROM THE BEGINNING.

All the conclusions about our lives—for those who chose to love Him—and God's intentions for us were decided and written down before time began.

HE FOLLOWED IT UP BY CALLING PEOPLE BY NAME.

And we choose whether we respond to that call or not. As Paul told Timothy, in 2 Timothy 1:9, that purpose and grace were given to those who were called. Therefore, **when we discover our purpose**, this is when we will also find the grace for accomplishing our mission.

HE SET THEM ON A SOLID BASIS WITH HIMSELF.

God set us in the one place where the covenant could never be broken: in Christ. Therefore, when He looks at us, He sees His Son, not our sin or failures.

AND THEN, AFTER GETTING THEM ESTABLISHED, HE STAYED WITH THEM TO THE END, GLORIOUSLY COMPLETING WHAT HE HAD BEGUN.

As Paul stated in Philippians 1:6, "*For I am* confident of this very thing, that He who began **a good work** in you will perfect it until the day of Christ Jesus."[197]

> God will never give up on you no matter how many times you may give up on yourself!

Where have you had an encounter with God's love or character that provokes some deep emotion in you?

_____
_____
_____
_____
_____
_____
_____

---

[197] New American Standard Bible 1995.

What emotion do you feel? Why do you think you felt this emotion?

How could this experience become a foundation for facing a future challenge (Goliath)?

BE PREPARED TO SHARE WITH YOUR GROUP YOUR ANSWERS TO THE QUESTIONS IN THIS CHAPTER.

CHAPTER 18
DEFINING MY NEW NORMAL

During this stage of our journey, on The Road Back Home, we learn to live as a new person in our normal world. As we say often at Pure Desire, we're not here to stop a behavior, but to change the way we do life.

This chapter is unique in that I don't have much reading for you to do. Instead—and this is far more challenging—I want you to apply all that we have learned so far. In completing this exercise, you will have a better understanding of your personal, God-given promises. You will have a much clearer comprehension of how your story ends! You will be able to see the limbic lies that are constantly at war in your head with the promises God has given you. This exercise will also help you describe the purpose of God in your life which is displayed in your prophetic promises!

> *You will never be able to find real freedom until you are able to identify the limbic lies that cause the pain in your life—these lies drive your addictive behavior. Therefore, not only must you identify each of these lies but bring the truth to confront each and every specific lie that cripples you.*
>
> DR. TED ROBERTS

#1. Identify the Limbic Lies You Face

Go back to Pillar 3, Lesson 1, in *Seven Pillars of Freedom* and read thoughtfully through the Ten Most Painful Moments in your life. Review them slowly in order to identify the limbic lie attached to the pain of that moment planted in your soul.

The lie may not be primarily in your conscious memory. The significant lies are usually like an iceberg with just the top of the lie breaking the surface of your conscious mind but the majority of its impact and power resides in your subconscious mind. Therefore, take some time and meditate on this assignment, asking the Holy Spirit to reveal to you the lies that you are battling with in your life. Ask Him to reveal the deep limbic lies that constantly drive your addictive behaviors below your conscious awareness.

Example:

Most Painful Moment: Getting yelled at by my dad and being told I would never amount to anything when I brought him the wrong tool.

Limbic Lie: I will always be rejected by others; I will never amount to anything.

Write down what you initially sense and observe in this exercise.

_____
_____
_____
_____
_____

Ask people who know you well what lies they sense you battling with in your life. (If married, start with your wife.)

_____
_____
_____
_____
_____

#2. List the Limbic Lies and the Possible Origin

Identify 3-4 limbic lies you are battling with and when you first believed the lie.

01. _____

I first believed this lie:

_____
_____
_____
_____

02. _____

I first believed this lie:

_____
_____
_____

03. _____

I first believed this lie:

_____
_____
_____

04. _____

I first believed this lie:

_____
_____
_____

#3. Your Attachment Style

How would you answer the following questions?

> When you were upset as a child what would you do? Think of a specific time you were hurt and what you did/how you responded as a child?

_____
_____
_____
_____

Are there any aspects from your early experiences that wounded you and resulted in you being set back? (i.e., set back: something hindered your ability to mature and move forward in life.)

_____
_____
_____
_____
_____
_____
_____

Is there anything in particular you learned from your childhood experiences?

_____
_____
_____
_____
_____
_____
_____

Identifying Your Attachment Style

When it comes to getting unstuck from trauma, it's important to recognize the role of attachment and how an insecure attachment or attachment injury may be contributing to our trauma.

Attachment refers to our ability to bond with others.[198] As infants, we depend on others to meet our needs and keep us safe. When our needs are consistently met in a safe environment, we tend to develop a secure attachment style. However, when our needs are neglected, and our environment feels scary and confusing, we are more likely to develop an insecure attachment style.

Our attachment style plays a significant role in how we relate to others in our adult relationships; not only intimate relationships, but all relationships. Our attachment

---

[198] Diane Poole Heller, *Understanding Attachment Styles and Their Effect on Relationships*, February 7, 2022, https://dianepooleheller.com/understanding-attachment-styles-and-their-effect-on-relationships/.

style reflects how we learned to be in relationships and forms the foundation for how we behave in relationships.

Based on research, several leading psychologists have determined that there are four types of attachment styles.[199] While this description is not exhaustive, it provides common characteristics found within each type.[200]

Secure:
- Easily developed relationships with others.
- Comfortable depending on others and being depended upon for support.
- Healthy balance between independence and connectedness.
- Relaxed, present, and playful in relationships.
- Practices repair; easily recovers from conflict.

Avoidant:
- Disconnected and closed-off in relationships.
- Lacks a sense of belonging.
- Finds intimate relationships distressing.
- Unable to emotionally connect.
- Prefers isolation.

Ambivalent:
- Craves connection, yet pushes others away.
- Fears abandonment and finds it difficult to trust others.
- Lacks self-care and the ability to self-soothe.
- Negatively misinterprets cues.
- Separation is distressing.

Disorganized:
- Wants close relationships, but fears it at the same time.
- Difficulty trusting others; views relationships as dangerous.
- Extreme dysregulation, often appearing chaotic.
- Acts out in confusing ways.
- Sudden mood shifts.

---

[199] Kendra Cherry, *What Is Attachment Theory? The Importance of Early Emotional Bonds*, Verywell Mind, July 17, 2019, https://www.verywellmind.com/what-is-attachment-theory-2795337.

[200] Diane Poole Heller, *Adult Attachment Styles Reference Guide*, Trauma Solutions, 2022.

Which of the four listed Attachment Styles best describes your response during your early childhood? Circle your response.

Secure   Avoidant   Ambivalent   Disorganized

Share a little about why you chose this Attachment Style to describe your response to experiences from your family of origin?

_____
_____
_____
_____

When looking at the characteristics of your Attachment Style, how might these characteristics reinforce the limbic lies you have believed about yourself?

_____
_____
_____

#4. Review Your Work from Pillar Five, Lesson Four

Seven Pillars of Freedom Workbook, page 189, 2021 version.

What three limbic lies did you list from this previous exercise?

01. _____
02. _____
03. _____

How do these three lies compare with the 3-4 lies identified in question #3 above?

_____
_____
_____

What prophetic promises are you using to defeat these limbic lies?

01. _____
02. _____
03. _____

#5. Review Your Three Circles

Seven Pillars of Freedom Workbook, page 188, 2021 version.

In **Seven Pillars of Freedom** you should have completed the Three Circles Relapse Prevention Tool. Take some time to review your Three Circles and add any new items to each circle as needed.

Next, I want you to do something brand new: add circles four and five! In circle five, boldly declare your God-given purpose in life. Why is this so important? Why are you alive?

I love Jay Stringer's research where he uncovered a powerful truth.

> "The greater a man's futility, the more likely he was to increase his pornography use. In fact, men were seven times more likely to escalate their pornography use if they lacked purpose in their lives."[201]
>
> JAY STRINGER, UNWANTED

Then, in circle four, list the goals you have in life because of your God-given purpose. How will you actually make a difference? What goals do you have in life in light of your God-given purpose? By listing your goals and consciously pursuing them, over time, you will develop the ability and inner strength to live out your true purpose.

When completed, this Five Circle Relapse Prevention Tool can become your "new normal" in life. This is a picture of the person you are called to be and the steps you will take to get there!

---

[201] Jay Stringer, *Unwanted: How Sexual Brokenness Reveals Our Way to Healing* (Colorado Springs: NavPress, 2018), 98.

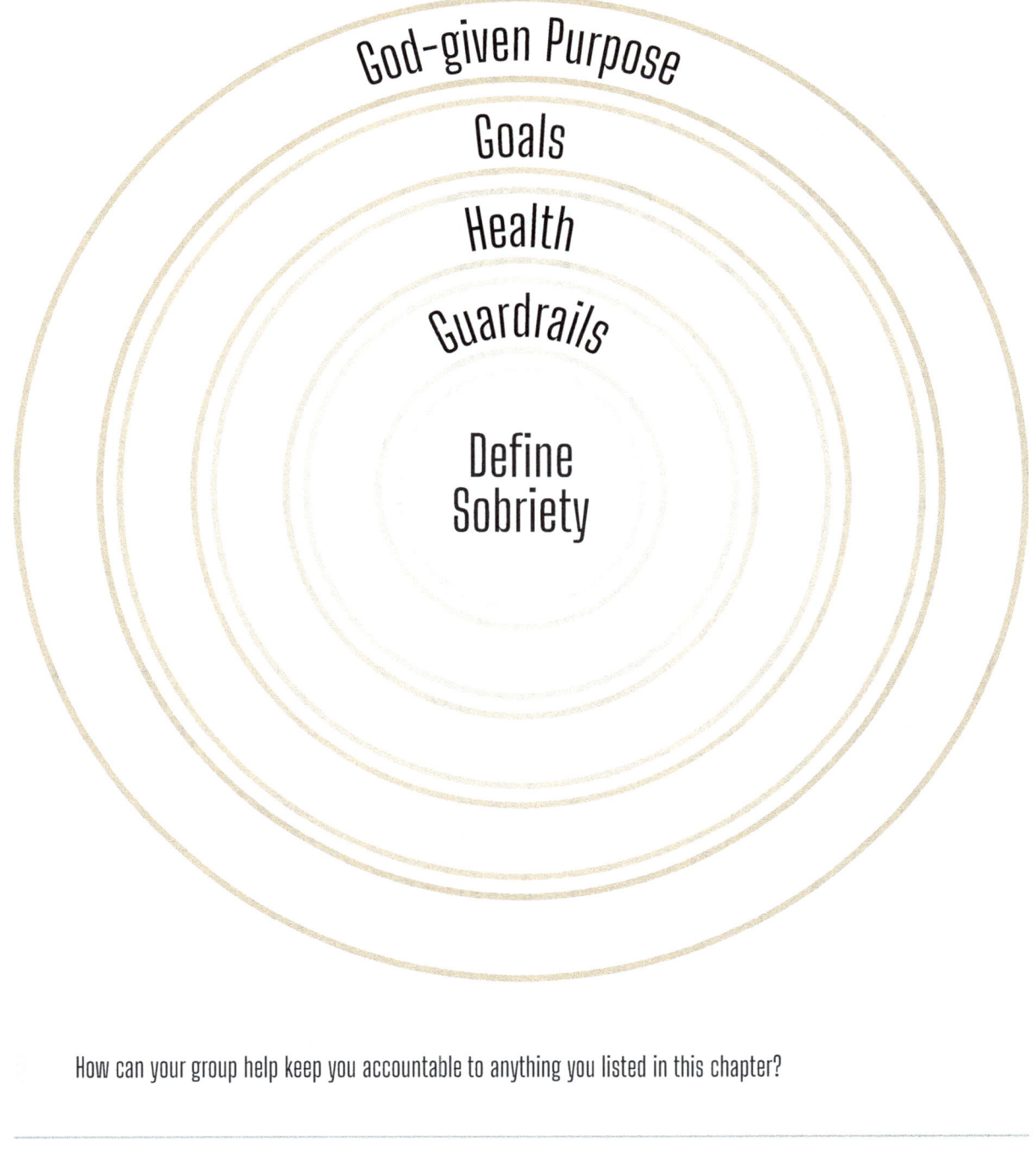

How can your group help keep you accountable to anything you listed in this chapter?

___

BE PREPARED TO SHARE WITH YOUR GROUP YOUR ANSWERS TO THE QUESTIONS IN THIS CHAPTER.

CHAPTER 19
STUMBLING INTO GREATNESS

Unlike Hollywood movies, being on The Road Back Home doesn't mean that the story ends and everyone lives "happily ever after." The truth is, as I mentioned in the introduction, we will walk our "...Way of the Warrior" pathway many times. The key question is, "How do we keep this from simply becoming one more cycle of highs and lows?"

A key to growth is learning the power of **lamenting**. Rather than running from fear, pain, or difficulty, the greatest skill we can learn is to take all of this to God. This is what the Bible calls lament, and in this chapter, we're going to look at how to lament well!

Some one-liners can haunt you long after you first hear them, like a small pebble that somehow ends up in your shoe. Initially, you hardly notice its presence, but slowly, almost imperceptibly, it takes on such a priority in your thought process that you can scarcely think of anything else!

After attending a seminar on Healthy Grieving and Loss presented by David Kessler, I suddenly realized King David's incredible wisdom.

Mr. Kessler made a statement I could not shake from my thinking. He was explaining a previous comment, "Death shapes grief," which suggests that the type of death your loved one suffered profoundly shapes your grief. For example, if your son died from a drug overdose, the grief would be very different compared to your son dying in an automotive accident. When a drug overdose is the cause of death, there is usually a lot of "If only..." battling going on in our head. "If only I had been more confrontational, he would be alive today!" "If only I had been more loving, he would be alive today!" We tend to treat ourselves harshly in grief, unlike the way we would treat a friend.

Here is the statement that haunted me for weeks: **Pain from loss is inevitable, but suffering is optional!** We often retraumatize ourselves in our grief. There is a significant difference between releasing grief and replaying traumatic events. King David was an expert at releasing his grief instead of attacking himself. **Unless we master his vital life skill, we can stay stuck in a death spiral of relapse.** A bit of paranoia can reside in all our souls because the future is unknown. The inconsistency of life can keep us all sitting on the edge of our chair, waiting for the next shoe to drop, or the next painful thing to impact our life.

Yet, as New Testament believers, we have a massive advantage in our struggles. The Cross of Christ gives us the ability to see God at work in our daily existence despite the inconsistencies of life. There is something declared at the Cross that is incredibly healing and hopeful. It is that which is always consistent, God Himself. He did battle with the inconsistencies in our broken world and the consistent won! Therefore, God is never frantically trying to figure out what to do with our evil world. He isn't caught off guard by the extent of our failures. This is precisely why one of my favorite one-liners is in the Gospel Mark 16:7:

> *"Now go and tell his disciples, and especially Peter, that he will go ahead of you to Galilee. You will see him there, just as he told you."*
> MARK 16:7 (CEV)

It was as if Christ could hardly wait to get out of the grave and send an encouraging word to Peter, "Tell Pete that he is next up to bat! It doesn't matter how many times he has struck out or stuck his foot in his mouth!" I think what makes it especially moving for me is that many scholars believe Mark drew his storyline from Peter.[202] I am sure when the old battle-scarred disciple dictated the memories of his days with the Savior, a tear or two ran down the side of his rugged face as he shared his personal experiences of Christ's passion for him. When Jesus said, "Make sure that Pete understands he has not struck out in life," these words of grace and encouragement were spoken to Peter despite the fact that he had painfully grieved the Master by his betrayal.

When I started reading through the Psalms of David, the thing that immediately grabbed my attention is how frequently he is complaining to God. He is expressing his frustrations about life through what is technically referred to as a lament; which is an intense expression of grief.[203] It is about praying while experiencing pain; and in David's imprecatory Psalms, you hear his rage expressed against his enemies.[204] He is not alone in his grieving. One out of every three Psalms are voiced in the minor key of lament, dealing with the agony of living in our broken world! Now initially, I thought David was complaining a lot to God, but I soon realized to pray in pain and to honestly struggle with the mess in our lives TAKES FAITH!

---

[202] David E. Garland, *The NIV Application Commentary: Mark* (Grand Rapids: Zondervan, 1996), 26-27.

[203] Walter C. Kaiser and Duane Garrett, *NIV Archaeological Study Bible* (Grand Rapids: Zondervan, 2006), 1304-6.

[204] Psalm 35:6 (NLT): "Make their [his enemies] path dark and slippery…" Psalm 58:6 (NIV): "Break the teeth in their mouths, O God;…" Psalm 108:13 "…he [God] will trample down our enemies."

It is far better than the silent treatment I give God at times. I end up living under the brutal lies that God doesn't care and He doesn't listen to me when I cry to Him in pain. Believing nothing can change, my silence is an expression of giving up! Turning to God and honestly expressing my doubts, questions, and hurts is one of the most profound and emotionally engaging demonstrations of my trust in God.

Joseph Campbell speaks of the ordeal the hero must go through as he faces the challenge of dealing with his deepest fears.

> **Where you stumble, there lies your treasure.**[205]

We see David stumbling into the greatness God had ordained for him to walk in! There are two places where David stumbled and almost lost everything. The first was obvious; his escapades with Bathsheba. The second was his total passivity with his son Absalom, which we looked at in depth in the last chapter.

Now here is an interesting question: what was the treasure David discovered in both of these spiritual face-plants? David had an amazing ability to grieve his mistakes and losses in life.

He knew how to pour out his pain and anguish to God in prayer. David knew how to lament his losses whether they were inflicted upon him by his enemies or they were a result of his own sinful choices. He understood the power of a lament which is found in a pain-filled prayer that ultimately leads to trust. It is the tear-stained pathway through the problem to the promise; from excruciating heartbreak to renewed hope.

I realized I had never learned the healing power of lamenting in my life. In Vietnam, I learned the classic response of a Marine if your wingman or flight leader "bought the farm" as we used to say; you got seriously drunk that night, sucked it up, and went on with the next day and dealt with the hangover. There is a huge problem with this approach. When you stuff your pain like this, it is only a matter of time before it rises up and bites you. This is especially true in your closet relationship, like in your marriage.

There is also a greater sense of freedom that comes to the human heart when you choose not to stuff your pain and keep moving forward. Grief is extremely powerful. It can grab a hold of your heart and refuse to let go. Therefore, instead of moving forward, you can remain stuck in your pain, anger, and depression. The turning point, from being embedded in your pain and anger to freedom, is if you can manage to find meaning in even the most senseless loss. **When everything appears to be at its worst and yet by the grace of God you find meaning, you will be at your best!**

---

[205] Diane K. Osbon, *Reflections on the Art of Living: A Joseph Campbell Companion* (New York: HarperCollins Publishers, 1991), 8, 24.

David was a master at finding meaning in his life despite the searing moments of pain he frequently dealt with in life. A classic example is the Song of the Bow which was the funeral song David composed for Saul and Jonathan.

> *Saul and Jonathan—beloved, beautiful! Together in life, together in death. Swifter than plummeting eagles, stronger than proud lions.*
>
> *O my dear brother Jonathan, I'm crushed by your death. Your friendship was a miracle-wonder, love far exceeding anything I've known—or ever hope to know.*
>
> 2 SAMUEL 1:23, 26 (MSG)

It is interesting to note that David wrote many laments concerning Saul's decade-long brutal campaign to find him and kill him. And Jonathan frequently saved his life during this crazy time in both their lives. After Jonathan's death, David found meaning and a way to sustain his love for Jonathan while he still moved forward in his life. This doesn't mean he stopped missing Jonathan. Instead, he experienced an increased awareness of just how precious he was to him. The love from Jonathan far exceeded anything he had known—or ever hoped to know.

David's words also describe how precious life is as well. We have no guarantee of how many days we have left. We may have many years ahead of us but what is always true is, when it ends, we rarely think life is long enough. Therefore, we must learn to value each day as a gift from God. This way, we will be living at our best.

All of us experience loss in life. Meaning is determined by our choosing to find life in the midst of pain and loss through the grace of God. Only we can discover what gives our life meaning. And meaningful connections will heal painful memories. The problem is, the only way we can avoid grief is by avoiding love. It's a package deal. If we love others, we will always face the risk of knowing sorrow. Meaning is the love David felt for Jonathan. Meaning is the way he chose to express gratitude to God for the gift of this person in his life.

Viktor Frankl, an Austrian psychiatrist and Holocaust survivor, wrote *Man's Search for Meaning*, depicting his struggle to find meaning while suffering through the indescribable hell of a Nazi concentration camp. Throughout his book, Frankl describes the insights he gained through unimaginable years of loss, suffering, and death. He wrote, "We who have lived in concentration camps can remember the men who walked through the huts comforting others, giving away their last piece of bread. They may have been few in number, but they offer sufficient proof that everything can be taken from a man but one thing: the last of the human freedoms—to choose one's attitude in any given set of circumstances, to choose one's own way."[206] Frankl learned, "When we are no longer able to change a situation...we are challenged

---

[206] Viktor Frankl, *Man's Search for Meaning* (Boston: Beacon Press, 2006), 66.

to change ourselves."²⁰⁷ When we make this choice, **we can turn tragedy into an occasion for growth**.

King David and the Psalms profoundly illustrate Frankl's observation: tragedy brings into our lives the challenge to change ourselves. But before we return to looking more in-depth at David's laments, let me ask you a few questions about your life experiences.

How good are you at grieving your losses in life? (e.g., I tend to stuff the pain and try to keep moving forward.)

_____
_____
_____
_____

Regarding your ability to grieve, circle what best fits you on this continuum:

Horrible   Struggling   Getting better   Move over David, I've got this!

Have you ever struggled with believing God is good in the midst of a personal tragedy in your life? Describe the nature of this loss and struggle in your life.

_____
_____
_____
_____

How did you finally come to walk in peace despite the pain? What was the turning point for you?

_____
_____
_____
_____

Usually, the grieving mind can't see much hope after loss. However, our failures and losses don't ever define us. This doesn't mean our grief will become smaller as time passes. It means, instead, **we must become bigger**!

---

²⁰⁷ Viktor Frankl, *Man's Search for Meaning*, 112.

An old Chinese proverb profoundly describes this dilemma: **The deepest pain has no words.** I have told my clients many times, "There will come a day when the memory of the loss will bring a smile to your face instead of a tear to your eyes." This is the process we all must go through with the Holy Spirit's help: first, the pain then meaning later.

David is continually walking through this same process in every one of his laments. The pattern of a biblical lament is evident as God leads the struggling believer on a journey. This poetic odyssey of the soul usually involves four elements:

01. an agonizing outcry to God,
02. an honest and often blunt complaint to God,
03. a request birthed out of personal pain, and
04. a statement of trust or praise.

Turning to God in prayer through a lament is one of the most costly and painful demonstrations of faith. It means you are usually praying for a solution and it is not working, YET. A lament is not a formula to get your prayers answered. It is a type of worship we naturally turn to when our pain level gets high enough because grief is never tame! It is how we can live amid such a broken world and still stay somewhat sane. Praying to God out of our pain is not so much a battle over the truth. Instead, it is about understanding how the painful emotions through the losses we have experienced end up feeling like the truth. But these painful emotions are never the final word. A lament is a messy way to pray.

This brings us to the next step in the process which we must learn; how to **BOLDLY** ask God. Our boldness in prayer is not based on our ego but on God's character. It is firmly built on who He is and what He has promised us. We must learn how to pray with boldness despite how we have been severely bruised by life. This is one of the tremendous benefits of laments. The trials of life can provoke us to reaffirm our absolute dependence on God. And laments provoke us to develop what I call "hard core patience." Trust is about talking with God and honestly sharing our pain-filled complaints with Him.

The turning point in every lament is found in words like **but, however, yet, or if**. For the simple reason that trust is not merely based on a belief or a conviction; it is trusting despite what the circumstances might lead us to believe. It is trusting despite what our feelings may be screaming at us right now! It is trusting what we know to be true even though the facts of our suffering may be calling everything else into question. Choosing to trust through lament demands we rejoice despite the fact that we have no idea how all of the pieces will ever fit together. At some point, we need to let God be the controller of our life; we need to take our hands off the steering wheel of our life and trust that somehow His gracious plan for our lives will work out—even if we have no idea how it will ever take place!

Augustine, the great leader of the early church, described the power of the Psalms of Lament:

> *The psalms are given to us as a divine pedagogy (a teaching tool) for our affections—God's way of reshaping our desires and perceptions so that they learn to lament the right things and take joy in the right things.*[208]

While lamenting can be a challenging journey, the good news is you don't have to walk alone! And when we are battling false limbic beliefs in our thinking, sometimes singing has the power to convince our emotions to change. This is especially true when we realize lamenting is a song we sing while living in a world that has been broken by sin. In Revelation, God gives us an exciting promise when Christ comes again:

> *"He will wipe away every tear from their eyes, and death shall be no more, neither shall there be mourning, nor crying, nor pain anymore, for the former things have passed away."*
> REVELATION 21:4 (ESV)

No one had to teach you how to cry. The moment you entered this broken world you instinctively knew how to do it. **However, the steps of lamenting must be learned.** It is how you make your way through the pain of living in a fallen world, while you tenaciously cling to the hope of the Gospel. It is how you live between the realities of tough times and God's incredible promises to you. Lamenting is a prayer in pain that leads to a new level of trust!

> " Show me how you lament
> and I will tell you who you are.[209]

For some, this exercise will be life-changing because it will start the journey to freedom you have sought for a long, long time. In the process of finally expressing yourself through a lament, you are going to discover WHO YOU ARE!

Why Lamenting Changes Us:

01. Your lament will put a spotlight on things in which you have placed too much hope—the idols in your life. The true test of idols in your life is how you respond to their loss.

02. Lamenting will point your heart toward the future victory God has set aside for you, through your tears you can realize Christ has yet to speak the final word.

---

[208] J. Todd Billings, *Rejoicing in Lament: Wrestling with Incurable Cancer and Life in Christ* (Grand Rapids: Brazos Press, 2015), 38.

[209] Author Unknown.

03. Your lament will uncover your deepest fears through your pain and, at the same time, anchor your heart to the truths you believe. Despite what you see, despite what you feel, despite what you may think, your song will affirm the truth that God's mercy is new to you each day!

04. Through your laments you will be able to live with pain beyond belief and discover God's sovereignty beyond your comprehension.

My Laments to God

Construct your laments using the biblical example as a template. I urge you, don't make this just a mental exercise. It will be a waste of time unless you answer the questions from your heart. If you make this exercise a right brain exercise, for some, the freedom you sought for years will finally come into view.

For some, I would recommend reading through David's Psalms for several days before you begin to construct your lament. For others, I would recommend spending several hours in meditation before you write your own lament. In LAMENT #1, I have written my personal lament in the left column as an example for you to follow. LAMENT #2 is for you to fill in.

LAMENT #1—EXAMPLE

Turn to God in the Struggle

O Lord, how long will you forget me? Forever? How long will you look the other way?

PSALM 13:1 (NLT)

Personal Lament

How long, O Lord, will I have to battle with Parkinson's disease?

The doctors constantly tell me "I will only get worse" and at times the pain is so crippling!

LAMENT #2—YOUR TURN

Turn to God in the Struggle

Lord, how many are my foes! How many rise up against me!

PSALM 3:1 (NIV)

Your Personal Lament

LAMENT #1—EXAMPLE	LAMENT #2—YOUR TURN
Complaint	**Your Complaint**
Turn and answer me, O Lord my God! Restore the sparkle to my eyes, or I will die.	*Many are saying of me, "God will not deliver him."*
PSALMS 13:3 (NLT)	PSALMS 3:2 (NIV)
Every day the battle only seems to get more intense! At times, I freeze up in public as if I am some kind of weirdo!	
O Lord, help me!	
Ask Boldly	**You Ask God Boldly**
Don't let my enemies gloat, saying, "We have defeated him!" Don't let them rejoice at my downfall.	*Deliver me, my God! Strike all my enemies on the jaw; break the teeth of the wicked.*
PSALMS 13:4 (NLT)	PSALMS 3:7 (NIV)
O Lord, You are my Shepherd and Healer. Let not Parkinson's **win this** battle—Your prophetic word to me was HEALING and I will not settle for anything less!	
Choose to Trust	**Your Choice to Trust**
But I trust in your unfailing love. I will rejoice because you have rescued me.	*But you, Lord, are a shield around me, my glory, the One who lifts my head high.* *I lay down and slept; I wake again because the Lord sustains me.*
PSALMS 13:5 (NLT)	PSALMS 3:3, 5 (NIV)
And I pray that You would open my eyes to see what You are doing in me. And who You are to me in this incredibly trying time that You never had the opportunity to be in my life before.	

I challenge you to take everything that is presently causing significant pain in your life and write a lament to the Lord concerning it. After you have finished with all of your laments to the Lord, look back over what you have written and answer the following questions.

> What idols did you uncover? (e.g., I realized my physical abilities were my idols; they were something that I relied upon for my self-esteem.)

> What victories lie ahead for you that Christ is yet to speak to? (e.g., Obviously, this is how Christ is going to fulfill His promise to me.)

> What fears do you see in your laments? (e.g., My fears were around whether or not Christ would come through for me.)

Where do you see God's sovereignty at work in your life?

_____

Seeing God's sovereignty at work in your life may be a very simple thing where after a time of reflection you suddenly realize God heard your lament and answered the cry of your troubled heart.

For me, freezing and being unable to move forward is one of the most embarrassing things that happen to me in public as a result of Parkinson's. When standing frozen before an open elevator door, I simply can't take a step forward! Recently, as I was visiting my neurologist at the Veterans hospital, I froze in the doorway to her office. She simply extended her foot in front of me and challenged me to step over it into her office. I immediately stepped boldly into her office! I didn't even recognize what had taken place. My wife sure did, and she now inserts her foot in front of me whenever I go into a freezing episode. I humorously tell her the reason I step so quickly forward is I know she will plant her foot in my rear end if I don't get moving! To me, this was God sovereignly answering my prayer on how to deal with this frustrating condition.

The nature of the promise God gave me with respect to my battle is this: "I will preserve you and give you as a covenant to the nations."[210] This promise came to me before I received a diagnosis of Parkinson's. I would have expected "I will heal you." But the nature of the promise illustrates God's sovereignty because it is obvious he knew I would be battling with a vicious disease. The miracle God is giving me is protecting me from experiencing a descent into dementia or an inability to move. God's healing power has sustained me and will sustain me for many years! My daily battle with this disease will give hope to many.

Your battle may be different from mine, but God has given you equally true promises. I pray that your life—your Way of the Warrior journey—will impact many lives around you!

Based on what you've learned, how is it helping you become a Compassionate Warrior? Be specific in your answer.

BE PREPARED TO SHARE WITH YOUR GROUP YOUR ANSWERS TO THE QUESTIONS IN THIS CHAPTER.

---

[210] Isaiah 49:8-10.

CONCLUSION
CLOSING COMMENTS

I have to admit I love the Eagles; they were one of the most successful bands of the 1970s. Their song *Desperado*[211] was never released as a single. Therefore it doesn't have much of a chart history. However, it is considered one of the Eagles' most celebrated songs. In fact, it was placed among Rolling Stone's "500 Greatest Songs of All Time."[212] It was also dubbed one of the "Top 100 Western Songs."[213] But the reason the song has been such a favorite of mine is connected to the past several decades of counseling guys struggling to get free from the deadly grip of sexual bondage. I find myself, almost unconsciously, rehearsing the words to myself as I help another guy try to get his thinking straight. The insights this song reveals into the addict's attitudes and blind spots are remarkable.

As I set out to write the final chapter of this book, which has taken almost five years of research and personal struggle to finish, I was trying to think of a way to review the overall content of all 20 chapters. I was primarily thinking of an individual who still might be losing the battle and feels hopeless. I wondered, *How can I help him see that his struggle isn't about having the necessary tools to get free?*

This book has all the tools you would ever need to enable you to get airborne. The problem doesn't lie in knowledge or lack of tools. **The problem lies in your limbic system, in the subconscious, or in the deeply rooted heart attitudes and/or blind spots.** For example, a client may be able to give an excellent analysis of his Arousal Template and a detailed explanation of why he does what he does, yet he continues to relapse again and again. This illustrates that you can't walk in sustained freedom by just getting your higher reasoning squared away. At some point in the process, you need to directly confront what I refer to as our "limbic cultural beliefs." Or, as the song *Desperado*[214] described it, you need to get free from your "cowboy thinking" to finally come home. You have been out ridin' fences for so long, you no longer even know the way back!

---

[211] Eagles, "*Desperado*." Track 5 on *Desperado*. Asylum Records, 1973, album.

[212] "The Rolling Stone's 500 Greatest Songs of All Time." *Rolling Stone*. Archived from the original on December 17, 2006.

[213] Western Writers of America, "The Top 100 Western Songs." *American Cowboy*. Archived from the original on 19 October 2010.

[214] Eagles, "*Desperado*."

Desperado
Why don't you come to your senses?
You've been out ridin' fences
For so long now
Oh, you're a hard one...[215]

The turning point in the story of the prodigal son took place when the wayward son "came to his senses."[216] It is fascinating that *Desperado*, which was written by Glenn Frey and Don Henley—who are not known as Christians—would start with such an apparent biblical reference. But I think the language of addiction is so universal that it is a way of expressing one's self that nearly everyone understands. It is the language of the common predicament of being an addict. And notice the results of sustained addiction on the human soul—"Oh, you're a hard one."[217] Why has the man become such a hard one? Because he has been out riding the fences so long, he isn't living for anything worth dying for! This is precisely why The Way of the Warrior is so important. Unless you find the Hero's Journey in your life, you will probably never be free. Instead, you will live a life of quiet desperation. In Luke 15:17, the phrase, "came to his senses" is so powerful! It helps the reader face the fact that he is struggling with something limbic in its origin. Addictions are always driven by your limbic system or as Paul so graphically described in Romans 7:15 (TPT):

"I'm a mystery to myself, for I want to do what is right, but end up doing what my moral instincts condemn."

Paul underlined the fact that decisions based on our limbic system alone don't make a bit of sense! They are clearly illogical if you pause for a moment and engage your prefrontal cortex. Your higher thinking process will quickly recognize that you just did STUPID!

The premiere example of what I am referring to was a past governor of New York, Eliot Spitzer. On March 10, 2008, *The New York Times* reported that Governor Eliot Spitzer had been caught arranging to meet with a high-end prostitute.[218] This formation was uncovered during a federal investigation. What makes the whole thing nuts is when you realize part of the reason Eliot Spitzer became the governor of New York. He became famous for busting Wall Street brokers for visiting high-priced prostitutes. So how did he get caught? The investigation of Spitzer was initiated after a report of suspicious transactions was made to the Treasury Department's Financial Crimes

---

[215] Eagles, "*Desperado*."

[216] Luke 15:17 (NIV).

[217] Eagles, "*Desperado*."

[218] Danny Hakim and William K. Rashbaum, "Spitzer Is Linked to Prostitution Ring," *The New York Times*, March 10, 2008, https://www.nytimes.com/2008/03/10/nyregion/10cnd-spitzer.html.

Enforcement Network. The technique of investigating suspicious transactions was the method Eliot used to catch the Wall Street brokers and it was the same technique the FBI used to catch him. Eliot Spitzer was forced to come to his senses!

> In what situations do you still find yourself doing "stupid?" Based on your work in this book and in this group, what is your remedy for this moving forward?

_____
_____
_____
_____
_____
_____
_____

> *But I know that you got your reasons*
> *These things that are pleasin' you*
> *Can hurt you somehow…*[219]

Notice where the song said you've "got your reasons." It didn't mean or imply your ideas make any sense! This is why lying or gaslighting can so quickly become part of your life. When you are a mystery to yourself as Paul expressed it, then lying swiftly becomes a lifestyle.

Chapter 6 looked at the men who surrounded David who eventually became his mighty men. You will never become who God has called you to become without your crew of men who are challenging your heart to line up with God's truth. Without a baseline of God's truth guiding your steps, you will find that the things which may be pleasing you, aren't just hurting you—in reality, they are killing you!

> *Don't you draw the queen of diamonds, boy*
> *She'll beat you if she's able*
> *You know the queen of hearts is always your best bet*
> *Now it seems to me some fine things*
> *Have been laid upon your table*
> *But you only want the ones that you can't get…*[220]

---

[219] Eagles, *"Desperado."*

[220] Eagles, *"Desperado."*

The *Desperado* way of thinking tends to view romantic relationships like a poker game—a game of chance. Somehow they didn't end up married to their "soulmate," but ended up with the queen of diamonds. I cannot tell you how many times I have heard a guy say something like, "I didn't marry the right lady; I have never been drawn to her!" They are expressing a common urban myth that their soulmate is out there somewhere and they need to find her. The problem is they chose the gal behind door number one, but hell is telling them they should have chosen door number three, where they would have found the queen of diamonds!

The truth is, you never marry the right person. You become the right person by what you go through together. You become soulmates through the adversities you face together. Remember, 69% of what you argue about as a couple, you will never resolve.[221] You will argue about it for the rest of your life! This is why, when you are in an argument, you desperately need to be right. This attitude is just plain stupid! Tom Robbins put it best when he said, "**We waste time looking for the perfect lover, instead of creating the perfect love.**"[222]

The lyrics of *Desperado* are an incredibly accurate description of what sexual addiction can do to your life. You will end up blind to the great blessing God has brought into your life—your wife. So many men I have counseled find themselves sexually unfulfilled in the relationship they have with their wife. The reason they find their wife unattractive is crystal clear. I simply tell them, "Here is the reason you will never get what you want: **you are trying to turn your wife into a porn queen**. God has given you this incredibly beautiful wife who has chosen to walk through hell with you. She is dealing with the searing pain of being betrayed at the most fundamental levels of her being. And she's decided to still take a risk in the relationship because of her God-given love for you. Yet you are still trying to run after some porn queen! This woman who always wants you and is always available, **she is pure fantasy and has never existed**. This is why you will always desire something you can never have."

In Chapter 4, you read the story of Curly's challenge of finding the "One Thing" in life, which he presents as the secret to life. The problem with Curley's challenge is that he's totally out of touch with his emotions, he lives on fantasies, and finds fulfillment primarily in his job. He is terrified of real intimacy. The words he shares with Billy Crystal in the movie *City Slickers*[223] gives us a vivid picture of how sexual addiction can lock you in a fantasy world that can never give you what you crave. It is the master strategy of hell!

---

[221] John Gottman and Nan Silver, *The Seven Principles for Making Marriage Work: Practical Guide from the Country's Foremost Relationship Expert* (New York: Harmony Books, 2015), 138.

[222] Sue Johnson and Kenneth Sanderfer, *Created for Connection: The "Hold Me Tight" Guide for Christian Couples* (New York: Hachette Book Group, 2016), 200.

[223] *City Slickers*, directed by Ron Underwood (Beverly Hills: Castle Rock Entertainment, 1991), film.

What steps are you taking now to create "the perfect love" in your marriage? If single, what steps are you taking to become a better husband or friend in the future?

_____

_____

_____

_____

Desperado
Oh, you ain't gettin' no younger
Your pain and your hunger
They're drivin' you home
And freedom, oh, freedom
Well that's just some people talking
Your prison is walking through this world all alone...[224]

The aging process is starting to catch up with him. It is slowly beginning to dawn on him: if something doesn't change in his life, he could end up being an old guy sitting in the corner still trapped in the binge/purge cycle—TOTALLY ALONE! The pain within is never silenced through medicating it or switching addictions. At this point in his life, he wonders if real freedom is ever possible for him. He has heard others talking about freedom, but he feels it is something that has never worked and will never work for him. It only further verifies that something is fundamentally wrong with him, deepening his sense of loneliness, isolation, and shame.

The only options left for him are living with an increased sense of sarcasm and jadedness toward life or just giving in to hopelessness. You never really experience God's grace and all of its incredible power until you come to the absolute end of yourself and are forced to make a **radical life-altering leap into God's grace**. This is why Chapters 7-9 are mandatory reading if you find yourself stuck and frustrated in life.

Don't your feet get cold in the wintertime?
The sky won't snow and the sun won't shine
It's hard to tell the night time from the day
You're losing all your highs and lows
Ain't it funny how the feeling goes
Away...[225]

---

[224] Eagles, "*Desperado.*"

[225] Eagles, "*Desperado.*"

Initially, we are drawn to addictions because they make us feel high. But it doesn't take too long before the high disappears. This is why we need to increase the dosage; it doesn't matter if we are talking about cocaine, sex, or booze. We increase the dosage TO FEEL NORMAL. Now we are caught in the death spiral of all addictions. Tolerance leads to an increased usage of the thing that is killing us as we try to feel NORMAL.[226] And soon, our feet are cold in the winter, and the sun doesn't shine, and it's hard to tell the nighttime from the day. We can find ourselves in seasons of despair, struggling to trust God.

The great warrior of the faith, Martin Luther, wrestled intensely with despair. Initially, it was so debilitating in his life that he would lock himself in his room for days. Then slowly, he came to realize that his despair was foundational for God to strengthen his faith. He said, "In an important sense, we **must despair** to wholeheartedly rely on Christ and what he has accomplished for us."[227] It causes us to abandon our self-reliance. Luther saw despair as the springboard to hope. Desperation looks around and sees the total absence of hope. Faith looks around and trusts that God is present and active, which always gives birth to hope.

Richard Rohr expresses this essential truth with the beautiful phrase: **EVERYTHING BELONGS**.[228] Having spiritual depth in our life is coming to the place where we see God as part of all things. He is at work in all circumstances, nothing is beyond the purposes of God. It doesn't matter if it will not snow or the sun will not shine. Holding on to hope while we battle with despair is KEY. We can't ignore the grief. We can't skip past despair. We need to feel to heal. The great saints of the faith saw sadness as a time of deepening our faith, a time of incubation and transformation. Yet **this critical, sacred space is the very space we are trying to avoid**. I like to put Paul's words into kind of a street translation of Romans 8:28:

We know that in all things, not just in the good things—even in the tough stuff, the depressing stuff, the awful things; the things that overwhelm us, knock us down, and cause us to despair—in everything, God is present, active, and working it out for our good! So get up: let's go and attack hell for a change!

How do we ever develop the ability to hold on to hope when we are fighting for our life in hand-to-hand combat with despair? Chapters 13 and 14 helped you face the challenge of dealing with the ordeal of the Inner Cave. The deepest despair we will ever deal with is when we lose hope in ourselves. In these impactful chapters, you were able to finally address the CRITIC WITHIN. Like Jim Carrey in *the Truman*

---

[226] Reef Karim and Priya Chaudhri, "Behavioral Addictions: An Overview," *Journal of Psychoactive Drugs*, 44 (1), 5–17, 2012, DOI: 10.1080/02791072.2012.662859.

[227] Kevin Cloud, *God and Hamilton: Spiritual Themes from the Life of Alexander Hamilton & the Broadway Musical He Inspired* (Sisters: Deep River Books, 2018), 147-174.

[228] Richard Rohr, *Everything Belongs: The Gift of Contemplative Prayer* (New York: The Crossroad Publishing Company, 2003), 33-34.

Show,[229] you confronted your deepest fears and discovered your way out of the false world by which you were entrapped. In Chapters 15 and 16, you uncovered the stunning power of the Resurrection of Jesus Christ. By this, I am not just referring to some vague theological truth. You realized why your betrayal of your wife through your addiction has crippled her so severely and why you can be so triggered by your teenage son's disrespect. In these chapters you discovered that Jesus **is far more humble than we are**! We remembered that Christ is the One with all the power, yet He allowed a minimum-wage Roman soldier to drive nails into His wrists and feet. He calls us to holiness yet defends a repentant hooker. How can we ever deal with a rebellious and trash-talking son? The same way God the Father dealt with you. He scandalously loved you through His son!

> What steps have you been taking to understand and address the critic within?

In Chapters 17, 18, and 19, we brought it all into a searing challenge that **pain from loss is inevitable, but suffering is optional**! King David broke every commandment God ever made, yet he finished his life to the applause of God the Father. And you wrote a lament like David did to process the pain and betrayals of your past. These chapters were absolutely foundational to breaking the power of relapse in your life. Resentments are extremely powerful in our lives. In the Big Book of Alcoholics Anonymous, resentments are identified as the NUMBER ONE CAUSE OF RELAPSE![230]

> *Desperado*
> *Why don't you come to your senses?*
> *Come down from your fences*
> *Open the gate*
> *It may be rainin'*
> *But there's a rainbow above you*
> *You better let somebody love you*
> *(Let somebody love you)*
> *You better let somebody love you*
> *Before it's too late*[231]

---

[229] *The Truman Show*, directed by Peter Weir (Hollywood: Paramount Pictures, 1998), film.

[230] Anonymous, *Alcoholics Anonymous: The Big Book*, 4th ed. (New York: Alcoholics Anonymous World Services, Inc., 2001).

[231] Eagles, "*Desperado*."

Notice how the fences have now become "your fences." These are the protective personalities you have developed through the years to guard against ever being hurt again. The truth is, the fences have become the walls of your jail cell—the personal prison you find yourself in now. The lifestyle of addiction has become a way of thinking and this way of relating to others has become a snare for you as you walk through this life. You feel TOTALLY ALONE at times. You feel like you are living in a permanent rainstorm and feel completely separated from God. You can't even recognize the rainbow of grace the Lord has placed over you. The song concludes with the haunting refrain: "... You better let somebody love you...better let somebody love you, before it is too late."[232]

What Does Too Late Look Like?

There is no question about it; in my opinion one of the saddest verses found in the Bible is Judges 16:20 (MSG):

Then she said, "The Philistines are on you, Samson!" He woke up, thinking, "I'll go out, like always, and shake free." He didn't realize that God had abandoned him.

I distinctly remember when I first read this translation—it shocked me! I couldn't believe it was possible to come to the place in your life where God would abandon you. Of course, it seems that Samson had never heard the word "moderation." Everything about him was extreme. It seems as if the Spirit of the Lord had painted the man as larger than life on the canvas of Scripture. He appears as a cross between Attila the Hun and Bozo the clown. In all the years I have spent listening to sermons or giving them, I don't think I have ever heard a positive sermon concerning Samson. I think the reason for this is, in his severe inclination to be impulsive and selfish, we see ourselves. And it scares us! Yet at the same time, there is something about the man that touches my heart. Maybe it's my military background coming out in me, but my soul is deeply touched when I read of him single-handedly taking on the Philistines.

Few men in life have had a better spiritual beginning. Samson was called by God from birth: "...and he shall **begin** to deliver Israel from the hands of the Philistines."[233] If deliverance had already begun, then Samson's ministry would not have been described as a beginning. By the very nature of the situation, Samson was called to fight alone. And it was an extremely difficult task because, at the time, the people of Israel had no ability to discern between good and evil. There was little difference between them and the world that surrounded them. Understanding the enormity of the task Samson faced helps us understand some of his erratic behavior—it doesn't condone his behavior but at least we can have some compassion toward him.

---

[232] Eagles, "*Desperado*."

[233] Judges 13:5 (NKJV).

In the last verse of Judges 15, an important truth appears giving us the context to understand Samson's point of failure: *"So he judged Israel twenty years in the days of the Philistines."*[234] For 20 years, he judged with peace and victory. It is fascinating to see how one verse of Scripture can so change a common misperception of an individual. Samson did not ricochet from one Philistine woman to another. He served Israel faithfully for 20 years. Yet, he was a man with a timebomb ticking away inside of him.

In Chapter 16, the time bomb detonates! It is as if we see, before our very own eyes, the total disintegration of a man of God. This incredible failure was not sudden or unexpected, for the infection of uncontrolled anger and lust had been eating at his soul for decades. As it explodes to the surface we see the depth of ugliness within Samson's heart. His uncontrolled anger and lust devoured the unique gifts God had given him from birth.

> *Samson went to Gaza and saw a prostitute. He went to her. The news got around: "Samson's here." They gathered around in hiding, waiting all night for him at the city gate, quiet as mice, thinking, "At sunrise we'll kill him."*
>
> JUDGES 16:1-2 (MSG)

The Philistine were sensing the impending disintegration of Samson. He had torn them a part for 20 years, yet they didn't hesitate to set up an ambush to destroy him. Why? They were sensing the smell of spiritual death in the air. One problem: Samson wakes up in the middle of the night and promptly tears the gates of the city off their hinges! In those days, the city gates were enormous, usually weighing several hundred pounds and were seen as a symbol of the city's power. He didn't just tear the city's gates off their hinges; he then dragged them all the way inland to Hebron.

Sin is a mocker. It will rise up with its Halloween mask on and jeer the person who thought he could sin and not have any consequences. But at some point, hell will come and collect its due. Samson had done what was right in his own eyes, but now the Philistines were going to viciously GOUGE OUT HIS EYES. The most expensive lessons we will ever learn in life are always about the consequences of sin.

This is exactly what too late looks like!

To the human eye, Samson is a wasted husk of a man. A bald buffoon characterization of what he once was. He is forced to dance before the Philistines like a trained monkey. He stands before them as a laughingstock. His garments are in tatters. His eyes empty sockets of shame. He smells of the dungeon. Behold the fool of Philistia! This is exactly where hell wants you to end up if you keep up your lifestyle of relapse.

---

[234] Judges 15:20 (NASB).

Here is good news in the pain of his failure: **Samson finally comes to know God**. This is the first time in his life we find him seeking God before he acts. We hear a prayer that has been refined by the pain of personal failure. A prayer of astonishing power because it is based on the character of God, not on Samson's frustrations.

Out of his pain and failures, he expresses his total commitment to God. Samson grabs the pillars of the temple of the Philistine god Dagon. And cries to God, *"Let me die with the Philistines!"*[235]

At that very moment, I can picture the Philistine rulers freezing in terror as they hear the groan of the collapsing roof over their heads. As they turn in horror, they see Samson once again transformed by the grace of God into a mighty warrior!

Judges 16 closes with a haunting epitaph: "So the dead whom he killed at his death were more than those whom he had killed during his life."[236] Samson rose above the dungeon. The grace of God transformed the prison of his mistakes. He became more than a conqueror in the fiercest battle anyone of us will ever face—being a total failure in the eyes of others. He finally confronted his deepest fears and responded to the challenge of the final words of the song *Desperado*. Our heavenly Father's love for us is so scandalous: we can be as messed up as Samson, but if we finally give up trying to control our world and reach out honestly to Him, acknowledge our desperate need for Him, then and there, **the crazy cycle of relapse will finally end in our life**!

> *You better let somebody love you*
> *Before it's too late*[237]

Samson finally lets God love him. And whenever this takes place in our lives, we become unstuck in life, and the relapses stop!

How do you think Samson's story applies to your life?

_____

_____

_____

_____

_____

_____

---

[235] Judges 16:30 (NLT).

[236] Judges 16:30 (ESV).

[237] Eagles, "*Desperado*."

How could you, like Samson, surrender ultimately to God's love in your life?

___

As we wrap up our study together, what will it look like for you to take divine revenge against the enemy? How will you use your story for God's glory?

___

Be sure to spend some time as a group praying over one another and the next steps God is calling each one of you to take.

Thank you so much for taking this journey with me on The Way of the Warrior. I trust God has used it to take you to new places in your journey. You were made to be a Compassionate Warrior! I am cheering you on every step of the way!

DR. T

What's Next For You?

Congratulations! You've completed all eight stages of the Hero's Journey! This may have been tough at times, challenging you beyond what you've experienced so far in your healing. And yet, here you are; ready to help others and serve them in a way you never before imagined. This is what becoming a Compassionate Warrior is all about—caring for others, walking alongside them on their journey, so they can experience the continued growth and healing you're now experiencing.

As you think about what comes next for you, consider these options:

- **Share your story.** You've done the work and found healing from your compulsive sexual behaviors. It's a story worth telling and will inspire others to find healing.
- **Become a group leader or coleader**, taking other men through *The Compassionate Warrior*.
- **Become a group leader or coleader** who wants to help men who are new to recovery begin their healing journey; first going through *Seven Pillars of Freedom* and then *The Compassionate Warrior*.
- **Talk to your church leadership** about starting Pure Desire groups at your church. Individual and Church Membership programs are available.
  - For individuals: https://puredesire.org/shop/individual-membership/
  - For churches: https://puredesire.org/shop/church-membership/

WHAT'S YOUR NEXT STEP?

Write down what's next for you. How has this journey to become a Compassionate Warrior inspired you? How do you plan to use your healing to help others?

_____
_____
_____
_____
_____
_____
_____

What's most important is that you do something: that you use your healing to help others. In your own family, among friends, and in your faith community there are people who need healing but don't know the way. You can help them find the hope and healing you've found.

You have what it takes to lead others to freedom—you are a Compassionate Warrior!

May God continue to bless your healing.

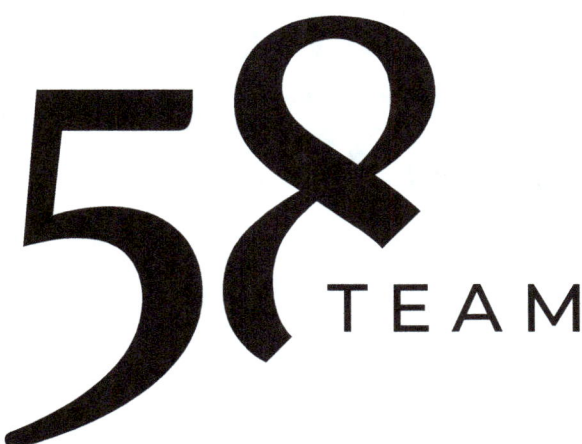

Has God used this journey through *The Compassionate Warrior* to change your future and your legacy? You can help others create their own legacy by joining Team 58!

Team 58 is a group of men and women dedicated to supporting Pure Desire through recurring monthly donations. They are passionate about advancing the message of hope and healing to people around the world.

Through ongoing, monthly support from people like you, we are able to expand the ministry and mission of Pure Desire: providing excellent counseling services, stellar group curriculum, and life-changing events.

As a Team 58 member, you'll receive up-to-date information on our latest ministry initiatives, exclusive invitations to meetings and events, and free Team 58 products.

To learn more about joining Team 58, visit **puredesire.org/give**.

Join Team 58 Today

AND BECOME A REBUILDER OF LIVES
AND RESTORER OF FAMILIES

CONTACT US

(503) 489-0230

info@puredesire.org

886 NW Corporate Drive, Troutdale, OR 97060

APPENDIX A
PRAYERS FOR BREAKING GENERATIONAL CURSES

When evening had come, they brought to Him many who were demon-possessed. And He cast out the spirits with a word, and healed all who were sick, that it might be fulfilled which was spoken by Isaiah the prophet, saying: "He Himself took our infirmities And bore our sicknesses."

MATTHEW 8:16-17 (NKJV)

Repeatedly, the New Testament makes such comments because looking back they came to grasp what would grant God the legal right to forgive and cleanse our sins and even sins of our forefathers. They realized that through Christ healing was available for those past, present, and even future sins. They were aware when Jesus died on the Cross declaring, "It is finished," everything necessary for healing was accomplished. There is nothing left that the enemy could use to prevent God's kids from experiencing God's healing touch in their life! The Cross was a verdict rendered. The Cross gave God the legal right to proclaim "Ted" as forgiven, even though I may not be able to articulate the specific sins or curses my forefathers may have released in my bloodline. The Cross also gave God the legal right to unleash health and wholeness to "Ted."

However, it is so crucial that we realize when Jesus cried out on the Cross "It is finished," it was a declaration of truth for all time. But a verdict declared if it is never acted on, has no power. It is legally the truth but if it is never acted on, it has no real authority in our life!

I think there are two areas where you will be confronting hell in the Courts of Heaven:

01. Places of personal responsibility

02. Places of generational vulnerability

The following two prayers are suggestions for the types of prayers you might want to learn and recite or put into your own words.

Personal Responsibility

Lord Jesus, my Savior, and Lord, I come before you laying my life at your feet. I want to become a living sacrifice for Your glory! I proclaim the fact that You are my Creator, and in You, I live and have my being. I am Yours and belong to You. I bring before You every word spoken about me that hell is presenting against me in the spirit realm, especially those words uttered by those who had authority over me and my life. I bring their words before You, O Sovereign Lord. First of all, I repent for every word spoken about me that was true, where I acted foolishly or disrespectfully.

I also repent of everything where I may have spoken evil of others. In both cases, I beseech you Jesus, my Savior, to forgive me because of Your shed blood that speaks for me now. I am genuinely sorry for the negative attitudes and harsh words I spoke against others who attacked me. I realize they were simply a reflection of the offender's own insecurities or pain. Lord, I am asking You to bless those who spoke ill against me. Bless the work of their hands, and I desire only good for them. That is why I am asking You not just to forgive me but to help me to see myself and others from Your perspective.

I ask that all the negative statements or words that hell has presented against me would be annulled, and the devil's accusations would be disqualified and rejected because of the cleansing power of Your shed blood and grace toward me. Now let the words they spoke against me be removed from the record of Heaven.

Let every voice raised against me be silenced by the Grace of God. I also ask that as You, Almighty God, declared in Psalms 139 verse 16, **"Your eyes saw my substance, being yet unformed. And in Your book they all were written, the days fashioned for me, when as yet there were none of them."** *Only allow what was written of me in my book in Heaven, to speak before Your courts. Only Your purposes concerning me are to be declared in Your courts. Finally, I ask because of Christ's blood, which was shed for me that Your healing power would flow into me and through me convincing others of Your love for them. I ask that Your prophetic promises which were spoken over me and were written about me in my book in Heaven, even before I was created, would take place. In Jesus' name, I pray. AMEN!*

Generational Vulnerabilities

(In this prayer, I personalized it from the traumatic moments from my family of origin. I would encourage you to do the same.)

Lord, I come before You today and proclaim the truth that I have been bought with a price, that Christ's death on the Cross purchased my total healing and freedom! Therefore, Judge of all the earth, as I enter Your courts, I repent of everything I have done even though You told me those things would hinder Your blessing and healing touch in my life. I heard Your voice but disregarded it. I repent of all rebellion in my life. I also repent of all and any rebellion in my bloodline. I don't know anything about the specifics of my bloodline because I was born out of wedlock. And I have never met my biological parents or any relatives, yet I sense a pull within that comes from deep inside me, rising against God. Therefore, I ask for Your forgiveness for me and my bloodline, I repent.

Lord Jesus, as You spoke to the woman in the Synagogue in Luke, chapter 13, I ask You to touch my life. **Luke declares the woman is bound**, *which means under an obligation of the law or duty. I have been tied up at times in my life by my own poor decisions or by a generational curse, which triggered a destructive reaction in me. I still remember the terrifying moment my stepfather attacked me for trying to protect my mother because he was drowning her. He violently hit me in the face knocking me into my room. As I struggled to get to my feet with blood pouring from my mouth, he threatened me with the statement, "If you get up again, I will kill you!" I made a decision that day not to get up. But out of a profound sense of injustice and rage, I pronounced a vow over my life, "I will never let another man treat me like that." I repent, Lord. I realize now that a VOW is nothing more than a self-curse. I spoke a curse of being condemned to a life of hyper-competition with every man I met for the next thirty years of my LIFE! I REPENT!*

As You spoke to the woman in the synagogue, I heard You declaring over me, **"You are set free, you are acquitted from your spirit of infirmity."** *I claim* **Colossians 2:14**. *I argue against hell and agree with heaven that the blood of Jesus removes every accusation against me. It even removes the self-curses I may have spoken over myself. The shed blood of Jesus is so powerful that the enemy can not use my own words against me in the Courts of Heaven. Your blood, Lord, removes everything that hell will ever use against me! That is the incredible power of Your grace. Jesus, I thank you for all You accomplished on the Cross for me! Thank you for the suffering You endured that provided legally for my total restoration and healing!* **For all eternity, I will stand in Your presence without sin or shame!** *AMEN!*

APPENDIX B
DEALING WITH ANGER

I hear so many complaints from men about how their wife can trigger an angry outburst from them. One of the most common scenarios is after the guy has been, in his opinion, doing everything he can. He hasn't acted out in a long time. He has done the hard recovery work faithfully every day. From his perspective, he has changed in some significant ways. And his wife can't see it; she will not trust him or affirm him for any of his hard work. She will not forgive him. These men often say, "She can't get free from the past!" They blow up and soon afterward, they relapse.

The vast majority of addicts I have counseled through the years were struggling with anger, which was the driving force behind their addictive behavior. Most men scored high on at least one of the four scales of Eroticized Rage on Sexual Dependency Inventory.[238] When I bring this to their attention, most are surprised and say, "But I am not angry." Their response indicates a profound misunderstanding of anger. They assumed the term refers to someone violently acting out like a predator. When rage and sex come together, it doesn't always have to express itself in physical violence.

A classic example was Darin, a client who was emotionally and physically abused by his dad for years.[239] He was also sexually abused by his older sister during his grade school years. His unresolved anger toward his family of origin was unconsciously expressed in his rage as an adult. He would compulsively seek the company of prostitutes and the sexual encounters were almost never characterized by physical violence. Many times, there was no sex involved. They would just sit and talk. This was, however, violent because of what was happening to his heart. He emotionally destroyed himself because no matter how many times he had promised himself he would never hire another prostitute, he found himself involved in the same crazy behavior again! He was taking his anger and pouring it on himself. This is also why his depression levels were so high and his self-esteem was so low. All of these facts were vividly affirmed by the combined tools we used in the clinical evaluation. For Darin, relapse had become a way of life.

---

[238] The Sexual Dependency Inventory is a powerful clinical tool developed by IITAP (International Institute of Trauma and Addiction Professional). I have every addicted client I counsel take this test. Along with the other tools we use, the PTSI-R and the Taylor-Johnson Temperament Analysis; I gain an understanding of what is driving their addictive behaviors.

[239] The individual's name was not Darin. The name has been changed to protect his confidentiality and the data presented is a combination of several clients I have helped.

For many addicts, identifying how anger is expressed through their sexual behavior is the critical first step in breaking the seemingly endless cycles of relapse. Learning how to process their unconscious anger in a healthy way is one of the more significant tasks of recovery!

Have you promised yourself and God, like Darin did for years: "I will never do that again?" Yet you continue to do the same crazy thing again!

What are some core limbic beliefs that lie at the root of your angry reactions in life? (e.g., No matter how hard I try, it will never be good enough; there is something fundamentally wrong with me.)

_____
_____
_____
_____

What are you really afraid of in life? (e.g., My sin being revealed; not being strong.)

_____
_____
_____
_____

What are your hot buttons in life? (e.g., Disrespected; not being listened to or ignored.)

_____
_____
_____
_____

I know these are very difficult questions to ask and answer. But if you don't have the courage to ask and answer them honestly, you will stay stuck in life. As a result, change won't happen and you will wound those who are closest to you, like your wife and kids, and the anger will only deepen.

We will automatically recreate the same type of home we grew up in, despite the fact that it drove us crazy, because it was programmed in our brain at a very early age.

You are reacting because of the pain of the past, rather than living in the present **and you do not even realize you are doing it**!

Why do we do this? Recent research has shown "that about 80% of the neural instructions for behavior are recorded in the implicit memory, outside our conscious awareness."[240] These behaviors are stabilized in our limbic brain by 18 months of age and continue to operate well into adulthood.

Here is the bottom line: your earliest learning can hijack the primary ways you react to the stressful times in life.[241] **You can't believe everything you think, especially in the midst of close personal conflicts!**

We can carry our family of origin around in our head and not even realize it. This is why Scripture challenges us to invite Jesus into our heart, not just our brain or mind. Biblically, our heart is best described as our limbic system.

We all have blind spots in our lives; therefore you are probably going to need some help from others to answer the following questions in depth. The guys in your group would be helpful, but you know who would be the best source of information? Your wife.

What are your hot buttons in life? (e.g., When I feel disrespected.) List your wife's responses to the same questions about you.

___

___

___

___

YOUR WIFE'S ANSWER:

___

___

___

___

What triggers your anger? What are you afraid of? (e.g., Fear of being "less than" or less of a man!)

___

___

___

___

---

[240] Alyson Quinn, *Experiential Unity Theory and Model: Treating Trauma in Therapy*, 2nd ed. (Blue Ridge Summit: Lexington Books, 2022), 69.

[241] Bremner, J D. "Does stress damage the brain?" *Biological Psychiatry* vol. 45,7 (1999): 797-805. doi:10.1016/s0006-3223(99)00009-8.

YOUR WIFE'S ANSWER:

_____
_____
_____
_____

What core limbic beliefs come from your past wounds and trigger you to live in the past rather than being present and trust God? (e.g., I am not enough; not strong enough; not smart enough.)

_____
_____
_____

YOUR WIFE'S ANSWER:

_____
_____
_____

The questions you have just dared to answer revealed where Exodus 20:5 is operating in your life. Do you remember what we discovered in Chapter 16: the biblical truth of generational curses? We are referring to skeletons from your past, left there by your dad or your grandmother or your great-aunt. In addition to this, there is the work of your first parents, Adam and Eve. Scripture is unambiguous. You were *in Adam when he broke God's commandment. We were condemned with him*.[242] But that's not the end of the story! Just as you were *in Adam* when he fell from Grace, so now, if you believe in Jesus, you are *in Christ* through faith. To remove the "generational curse" you have to be grafted into a whole new family tree.[243]

We must understand this will always involve a choice on our part. As pointed out in the previous chapter, generational curses are not set in stone. We are not talking about an irreversible "curse." Spiritual deliverance is available to everyone who sincerely calls upon the name of the Lord.[244] In order to honestly call upon the Lord, we must understand what is provoking us to act in such a destructive way. We cannot change what we don't understand.

---

[242] Romans 5:12 (NIRV).
[243] Romans 11:11-24 (NIRV).
[244] Romans 11:13 (NIRV).

ABOUT THE AUTHORS

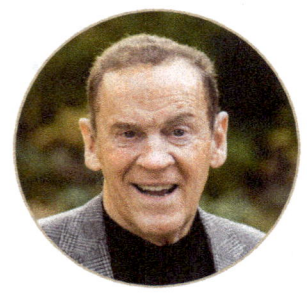

Dr. Ted Roberts

Dr. Ted Roberts is a Pastoral Sex Addiction Professional (PSAP) and a Pastoral Multiple Addiction Professional (PMAP) through the International Institute for Trauma and Addiction Professionals (IITAP). He is trained in the use of Brainspotting: a powerful, focused treatment method that works by identifying, processing, and releasing core neurophysiological sources of emotional and body pain, trauma, dissociation, and a variety of other challenging symptoms.

As the senior pastor of East Hill Church for more than 25 years, he counseled many men struggling with sexual bondage. Recognizing the seriousness of unhealthy sexual behaviors in the church and the limited resources available in the Christian arena, he worked with Dr. Patrick Carnes to develop the Seven Pillars to Freedom Workbook. This resource, biblically based and clinically informed, was instrumental in helping men and women find freedom from sexually destructive behaviors.

In 2007, Dr. Ted resigned as the senior pastor, took a leap of faith, and founded Pure Desire Ministries International.

Dr. Ted has worked with clients of all ages, both individuals and couples, who struggle with sexual and love addiction, same-sex attraction, betrayal, and much more. He feels uniquely called to help pastors who are experiencing sexual bondage and shame, which has a profound effect on their calling in the church.

Dr. Ted is passionate about helping people who have suffered pain and trauma in their lives, feeling privileged to observe major miracles in their lives as they find lifelong healing through Pure Desire.

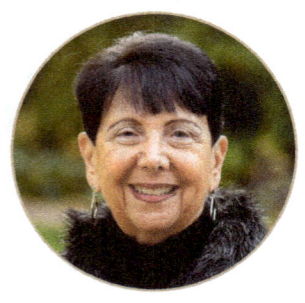

Diane Roberts

Diane Roberts is a licensed pastor and IITAP certified PSAP counselor with more than 30 years experience in ministry, counseling women, developing curriculum for healing, and training leaders. Her training and experience as a teacher provided a strong knowledge base for curriculum development.

In the early 1990s, she and her husband, Ted, recognized a growing issue with unhealthy sexual behaviors in the church. Based on Dr. Patrick Carnes research, she was instrumental in developing curriculum to facilitate sexual healing in the church.

In 2007, Diane cofounded Pure Desire Ministries International. With a pastoral background, Diane has worked with women who struggle with betrayal and trauma, helping them establish safety and set healthy boundaries. Alongside her husband, she has counseled couples who are experiencing the aftermath of sexual addiction and betrayal, helping them find restoration in their marriage.

Diane enjoys bringing a holistic approach to healing, using clinical tools that combine a scientific understanding of addiction, trauma, and the brain with a biblical foundation. She is honored to witness how the Holy Spirit provides a supernatural understanding and uses her as a vessel to bring health and wholeness to the lives of individuals and couples through Pure Desire.

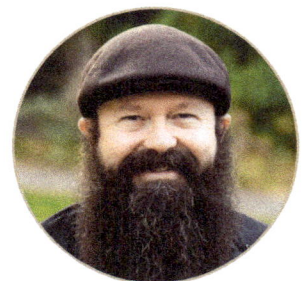

Robert Vander Meer

Robert Vander Meer has a passion for the field of sexual addiction as a result of his own addiction and recovery. Everything he does is a result of the recovery journey he has been on. It's not over, but continuing, and will continue the rest of his life.

Robert has vast ministry experience including being a Foursquare Pastor, Lead Pastor, Associate Pastor, Co-Pastor, and College Pastor. He has been a Clinician and groups facilitator with Pure Desire for the last 12 years. Robert is a frequent podcast guest, blog author, resource contributor, and often one of the mainstage speakers at Pure Desire events. In addition, he is a certified Pastoral Sex Addiction Professional-Supervisor through IITAP (International Institute for Trauma and Addiction Professionals).

Helping himself and others find value in their unique identity is one of the ways he has seen the Lord show up in his life and in the lives of others. In this unique identity, he and others have been able to engage in relationships in a new way. This is where all have found that they can continue in this healing journey most effectively as ourselves, that who we are is wanted, valuable, and loved. Life isn't easy but it's easier when we can be honest and vulnerable with people we have learned to trust.